ID0622885

The

Fasting Path

Other Books by Stephen Harrod Buhner

Vital Man: Natural Health Care for Men at Midlife

*The Lost Language of Plants: The Ecological Importance
of Plant Medicines for Life on Earth*

Herbs for Hepatitis C and the Liver

*Herbal Antibiotics: Natural Alternatives for
Drug-Resistant Bacteria*

*Sacred and Herbal Healing Beers:
The Secrets of Ancient Fermentation*

One Spirit, Many Peoples: A Manifesto for Earth Spirituality

*Sacred Plant Medicine: Explorations in
the Practice of Indigenous Herbalism*

The
Fasting Path

The Way to Spiritual, Physical, and
Emotional Enlightenment

Stephen Harrod Buhner

Avery

a member of

Penguin Group (USA) Inc.

New York   2003

Neither the publisher nor the author is engaged in rendering professional advice or services to the individual reader. The ideas, procedures, and suggestions contained in this book are not intended as a substitute for consulting with your physician. All matters regarding health require medical supervision. Neither the author nor the publisher shall be liable or responsible for any loss, injury, or damage allegedly arising from any information or suggestion in this book. The opinions expressed in this book represent the personal views of the author and not of the publisher.

The recipes in this book are to be followed exactly as written. Neither the publisher nor the author is responsible for your specific health or allergy needs that may require medical supervision, or for any adverse reactions to the recipes contained in this book.

While the author has made every effort to provide accurate telephone numbers and Internet addresses at the time of publication, neither the publisher nor the author assumes any responsibility for errors or for changes that occur after publication.

Most Avery books are available at special quantity discounts for bulk purchase for sales promotions, premiums, fund-raising, and educational needs. Special books or book excerpts also can be created to fit specific needs. For details, write Penguin Group (USA) Inc. Special Markets, 375 Hudson Street, New York, NY 10014.

Final stanza of "A Ritual to Read to Each Other" copyright 1960, 1998 by the estate of William Stafford. Reprinted from *The Way It Is: New and Selected Poems* with the permission of Graywolf Press, Saint Paul, Minnesota.

Excerpts from *When Food Is Love* by Geneen Roth copyright © 1991 by Geneen Roth. Used by permission of Dutton, a member of Penguin Group (USA) Inc.

"Oracles" by Dale Pendell reprinted with permission.

a member of
Penguin Group (USA) Inc.
375 Hudson Street
New York, NY 10014
www.penguin.com

Copyright © 2003 by Stephen Harrod Buhner
All rights reserved. This book, or parts thereof, may not
be reproduced in any form without permission.
Published simultaneously in Canada

Library of Congress Cataloging-in-Publication Data

Buhner, Stephen Harrod.
The fasting path : the way to spiritual, physical,
and emotional enlightenment / Stephen Harrod Buhner.
p. cm.
Includes bibliographical references and index.
ISBN 1-58333-170-0
1. Fasting. 2. Fasting—Therapeutic use. 3. Detoxification (Health). I. Title.
BV5055.B85 2003   2003045352
613.2'5—dc21

Printed in the United States of America
1   3   5   7   9   10   8   6   4   2

Book design by Meighan Cavanaugh

For all those who labor in interior time

Acknowledgments

Trishuwa, who helped when I could find no light at the end of the tunnel; the women who have traveled in darkness learning how to restore the human sanctity of the body, including Geneen Roth, Carol Normandi, and Laurelee Roark; and as always, Robert Bly and James Hillman.

Contents

Preface

Fast: to keep, bind, observe, pledge. Firmly, fixedly, closely, quickly, to attach. From the Gothic fastan, *which is the root used in nearly all northern European languages for the word* fast.

—OXFORD ENGLISH DICTIONARY

Throughout the habitation of our species on this planet, fasting has, until our time, been concerned with much more than the physical body. Traditionally, fasting concerned itself with the emotions—our psychological selves—and with the soul and our souls' communication with the sacred. Because of unique historical events that have taken place over the past five hundred years, the focus of fasting has shifted—either to the body's health alone or to a drive to subdue the body in order to conquer the "evils" (or limitations) of the flesh. Neither of these perspectives are of much interest to me—except in how they affect contemporary approaches to the more ancient and holistic fasting that our species has always known.

You *can* use this book to explore *only* the spiritual aspects of fasting, or *only* the emotional aspects of fasting, or *only* the physical aspects of fasting. All are examined in the pages that follow. Doing so will still be of benefit to you. But fasting is really a highly complex and multifaceted act that is most effective when viewed as a whole and not as a mix of three pieces glued together. For when we fast we are engaging in a multidimensional process filled with myriad ramifications for who we are and how we live. What we are doing is deciding to consciously engage the hidden parts of ourselves, the secret face of the sacred that is within all forms of the material world, and our most fundamental relationships with food and nurturing.

When we decide to fast we make the choice to become aware.

A Note to the Reader: About Water and Juice Fasting

Although many fasting proponents insist that a true fast allows only water, in actual fact fasting means the intake of nothing at all. While it is commonly believed that water is necessary during fasting, this is not actually so. During the powerful fasting movements of the late nineteenth century, physicians carried out a number of very sophisticated, controlled studies of the physical dynamics of fasting. Their research, most of which was published by the Carnegie Institute in Washington, D.C., is highly provocative and intriguing. A number of the fasters they studied took no food *or* water for as long as 15 days, then took water only for up to another 30 days. They were under a physician's care daily, their vital signs closely monitored. None of them experienced any physically detrimental effects from fasting without water.

Nonwater fasting is highly unusual now; the only instances I know of are during certain types of vision quests. Currently, the most common forms of fasting are water and juice fasts. (Juice fasts, for me, also include lemonade/maple syrup and herbal tea fasts.) There is, however, a significant difference between the physical impacts of these two types of fasts. A water fast is more demanding and is accompanied by tremendous fatigue. It is not possible to work a regular schedule on a water fast. Physical exercise is difficult; usually easy walks are the most that is possible. A juice fast possesses many of the benefits of water fasting but is less intense; energy levels remain high, and work and exercise are still possible. Both have their benefits.

Water fasting is indicated for those who are working with more serious or long-term chronic conditions, wish to lose a large amount of weight, or desire to engage in deep transformational fasting. Juice fasting is especially good for regular tuneups of the body, for initial fasting work, or if you cannot arrange time off from work and still wish to fast. Historically, wilderness fasting retreats or vision quests are almost exclusively water fasts.

Although most people can safely fast, there are a few who, because of special conditions, should not. Read pages 100–102 to determine whether or not it is safe for you to undertake a fast. Consult a health-care professional before beginning a fast for the first time, to ensure that you are in good health.

For it is important that awake people be awake,
or a breaking line may discourage them back to sleep;
the signals we give—yes, or no, or maybe—
should be clear: the darkness around us is deep.

—WILLIAM STAFFORD,

"A RITUAL TO READ TO EACH OTHER"

1

On Fasting and the Spiritual Life

When we fight for the soul and its life, we receive as reward
not fame, not wages, not friends, but what is already in the
soul, a freshness that no one can destroy.

— ROBERT BLY

What the eyes are for the outer world, fasts are for the inner.

— GANDHI

There is an old Native American observation that when the
white man took tobacco back to the Old World he merely took its
body—its spirit was left in North America, lying on the ground.
Tobacco, for ancient peoples, was considered a holy plant, a plant

with great spiritual powers, whose purpose was to facilitate communication between human beings and the sacred powers of the Earth and Universe. This same dynamic, the splitting apart of the body and the spirit of a thing, has occurred with a great many other things that have always been considered intrinsically spiritual in nature. Fasting is one of them.

For the past five hundred years the trend has been, increasingly, to view matter as devoid of spirit, intelligence, soul, or purpose. A lump of rock—merely inanimate matter, a resource or something on which to stub your toe, certainly not something filled with soul. But throughout human history, human cultural perspectives about such things have been very different. In earlier times, it was commonly understood, irrespective of culture or historical period, that the world was alive, that all things possessed souls, that human beings were only one of a multitude of ensouled beings, and that there was a constant soul energy going out of and into our bodies as we traveled through the world. Beyond any health aspects it was known to possess, fasting, like tobacco, was one way, an important way, to deepen communication with the sacred. Fasting, it was recognized, increased human sensitivity to the nonmaterial world, enhanced personal experience of the sacredness of both self and Universe, and helped the fasting person regain a sense of orientation and purpose.

Compared to the mechanistic worldview that is now so dominant, older perspectives of the Universe are much more complex and multidimensional. Ancient and nonindustrial cultures understood that the Universe and the Earth were deeply sacred. Human beings, along with all other life forms, are, within those earlier perspectives, considered to be inextricably embedded in this sacred world, indeed to be an integral part of it. These ancient viewpoints are not *beliefs* as we now understand the term but are representative of a living experience. They lie deep within the epistemology—the way people see reality—of all older cultures. Their components are remarkably similar in all cultures on all continents and in all times. While containing numerous variations, themes, and differences, they do have a basic framework that is very similar in a number of areas. Most assert the following.

1. At the center of all things is spirit. In other words, there is a central underlying unifying force in the Universe that is sacred in nature.
2. All matter is made from this substance. In other words, the sacred manifests itself in physical form.
3. Because all matter is made from the sacred, all things possess a soul, a sacred intelligence, or *logos*.
4. Because human beings are generated out of this same substance, it is possible for human beings to communicate with the soul or intelligence in all other matter and for those intelligences to communicate with human beings.
5. Human beings were ignorant when they arrived here, and the powers of the Earth and the various intelligences in all things began to teach them how to be human. This is still true. It is not possible for new generations to become human without this communication or teaching from the natural world.
6. Parts of the Earth can manifest more or less sacredness, just like human beings. A human being can never know when some part of the Earth might begin expressing deep levels of sacredness or begin talking to him or her. Therefore it is important to cultivate attentiveness of mind.

7. Human beings are only one of the many life forms of
the Earth, neither more nor less important than the
others. Failure to remember this can be catastrophic
for individuals, nations, and peoples.

Luther Standing Bear, a Sioux holy man, writing in the early
twentieth century, gives a typical description of this way of experiencing the world:

From Wakan Tanka, the Great Spirit, there came a great
unifying force that flowed in and through all things—the
flowers of the plains, blowing wind, rocks, trees, birds,
animals—and was the same force that had been breathed
into the first man. Thus all things were kindred, and
were brought together by the same Great Mystery.[1]

These ancient perspectives, in a very rough way, represent,
perhaps, the oldest epistemology of humankind and have been
present in most cultures on Earth. Each one has codified this in
differing ways, described it in different words, rigidified it as religion in varying forms. But beyond its varying forms of expression
in different cultures and beyond its classification as religion it represents a specific kind of human relationship with a living, aware,
and sacred Universe and Earth.

For ancient peoples, human beings were never alone; there
was a continual exchange of soul essence between people and the
other inhabitants of Earth, a constant, intimate sharing of life
essence between life forms that are, at their core, kin. Something
was leaving their bodies and something entering them. Perhaps
the easiest way to gain a contemporary sense of this experience is if
you think about puppies, if you, perhaps, imagine a puppy slowly

walking across the floor in front of you now. His nose is to the floor, completely caught up in what he is smelling. His hind legs are walking a bit faster than his front legs, so his body is walking at that slight angle at which puppies often walk. His tail is up, slowly waving back and forth as he concentrates on what he is smelling. You can stand it no longer, and so you say, "Here, boy, come on, here." And perhaps you pat your leg. The puppy looks up and sees you and stops; his eyes light up in excitement, his body turns to you, and all of his energy says, "It's you! It's you! I have been looking everywhere for you!" At that moment you can feel something leave the puppy's body and enter yours, and something leaves your body and enters the puppy's, and the two of you want nothing more than to touch each other. You pick him up, running your hands over his back and sides, petting his head, and perhaps he licks your hands or face, and both of you feel a particular kind of feeling. A very good, warm feeling.

(If you have ever seen a puppy encounter someone who does not like puppies, who does not send something out of his or her body to the puppy, you have seen what puppies generally do in response—they respond to that person with caution, sometimes with active dislike.)

This kind of exchange with a puppy is one of the most satisfying experiences we can have as human beings. We experience it when we see old friends we love, or close family, or a beloved pet. It's as real as a lightning strike or the kiss of one's beloved, yet there is no word in our language for it, this exchange of soul essence. *Love,* that overworked word, is not really descriptive of what is happening. There is, for a moment, a common meeting of similarly inclined souls, an exchange of something essential, a touching that goes much deeper than the physical. It is one of the most meaningful experiences we can know as human beings, and once upon a time all human beings knew of it, named it, and experienced it—not only with family, friends, and pets but with all of creation. For it was known that all things are alive and filled with soul and purpose and intelligence and that this type of sharing can take place anytime, with anything—anything at all.

But in our modern drive to reduce the Universe to a collection of parts, to dissect and study it, something crucial has been lost; and, increasingly, people are finding something amiss in seeing the world as merely inanimate matter. Two very important aspects of human experience stand out as having been severely diminished by the assumption that there is no sacredness and aliveness in the world: the complexity of feeling that it is possible for human beings to develop, and deep, daily connection with the sacred.

These two things are crucial to understand when exploring the deeper aspects of fasting, for fasting increases human sensitivity to just these things. Spiritual fasting is, above all else, a way to encounter the deeper spiritual world directly, to explore its territory, and to bring back a knowledge essential to living a fulfilled life.

The Sacred and the Heart

All ancient and nonindustrial cultures make an interesting assertion: that the soul and its intelligence are located around or in the heart. Further, it is this heart intelligence that directly experiences the deep spiritual realities embedded within the world. This understanding is crucial to transformational fasting. During deep fasting, what is called the rational mind is left behind for a time, and a different intelligence, located in the heart, is activated. During such fasts, reliance on two-dimensional sight begins to weaken, there is a thinning of the wall between us and all other things, and the organ of perception uniquely designed to perceive the sacred, the heart, begins to take on more and more importance. As deep fasts progress, as the veil between us and the spiritual world thins, the heart begins to perceive the hidden face of the sacred within everyday things.

Each thing of the world possesses a hidden aspect. This is not hidden in the sense that it is intentionally concealed but in that it must be seen with other eyes than the physical. Physical sight is, in many respects, only a two-dimensional sight. Things that exist outside of that plane of two-dimensional vision cannot be seen, no matter how hard one tries, if only the physical eyes are used. Like many things, sight possesses both emotional and spiritual dimensions. These more sophisticated elements of sight have to be cultivated, however, and the skill to use them must be developed over time. There is nothing necessarily grandiose about this. It is a simple thing, a natural part of the human journey, a potential skill that belongs to each of us by birthright. One does not need to be

> The heart brings us authentic tidings of invisible things.
>
> —JAMES HILLMAN

especially pure or spiritual, to find a master or a guru, or to be born with special talents in order to develop this deeper way of seeing. The understanding that physical vision is only the beginning of the complexity that is *sight* is, however, an important initial step. Once this is recognized, when the deeper elements of sight manifest, as they naturally do during life, the skill of seeing can be intentionally cultivated. And the organ through which the hidden aspects of the physical world are apprehended is the heart. While modern science generally insists that the heart is only a muscular pump, it is also true that there are more than forty thousand sensory neurons in the heart, the same kind of neurons that are found in the brain.

Each individual section of the brain contains thousands to millions of neurons, several billion when all added together. Significantly, certain crucial subcortical centers of the brain contain the same number of neurons as the heart. The heart possesses its own nervous system and, in essence, actually *is* a specialized brain that processes specific types of information. The heart is tightly interwoven into the neurophysiology of the brain, interconnected with the amygdala, thalamus, and cortex.

These three brain centers are primarily concerned with (1) emotional memories and processing; (2) sensory experience; and (3) problem solving, reasoning, and learning. What this means is that our *experience* of the world is routed first through our heart, which "thinks" about the experience and then sends the data to the brain for further processing. When the heart receives information back from the brain about how to respond, the heart analyzes it and decides whether or not the actions the brain wants to take are going to be effective. There is a neural dialogue between the heart and brain, and in essence the two decide together what to do. While the brain can and does do a great many things with the information it receives, the heart can override it, directing and controlling behavior if it decides to do so. Knowledge about these deeper aspects of the heart has, throughout history, been held by all of the world's cultures.

Our daily language contains (as do all languages) wisdom

about the heart that we rarely call up into our conscious minds. We have all known, at one time or another, a man who is "big-hearted" or a woman who is "goodhearted" or have even had friends who are "kindhearted." If we tell them so, we may do it in a "heart-felt" way. We sometimes eat a "hearty" meal, share a "hearty" laugh, or even look "hearty." Our profession or our mate may become the "heart" of our life, or we may work for long years to attain our "heart's desire." And because the heart does in fact act as a specialized brain, it is actually possible to "follow your heart" or to "listen to your heart."

If we are dejected or hopeless, it may be said that we have "lost heart." If a loved one rejects us, we can become "broken-hearted." If we are being unkind, someone may implore us to "have a heart" or not be "heartless." People can be "coldhearted" and cruel, and it is literally possible to be "hardhearted." During arteriosclerosis, or hardening of the arteries, bony calcium growths can form in the openings to the heart and occlude blood flow. These growths can become stone hard, hard enough to break saws specially designed to cut through bone.

Over the past twenty years, researchers in an emerging specialty, neurocardiology, have discovered that the heart really is a specialized brain in its own right. It can feel, sense, learn, and re-member (as Balzac noted some 150 years ago when he said that the heart has its own memory). As the heart senses the world outside us it generates emotions in response to the type of informa-tion or the meanings embedded within the information that we are receiving. These emotional complexes that are generated are the linguistics of the heart. They are sophisticated informational cues or gestalts about the world around us and can be extremely complicated. Emotional languaging is very different from lan-guages built around words. The latter tend to be handled more linearly (two-dimensional processing), while the emotional language of the heart is handled more intuitively (three-dimensional processing).

Many of the emotional experiences that flow through the heart are stored as memories within the heart, much as memories are stored in the brain. The heart literally learns from the emotional experiences it has and begins to act in certain ways on the basis of what it learns. It begins producing different hormones and creating different beating patterns depending on what experiences flow through it and what it decides about those experiences.

> The evisceration of tradition takes place when the heart loses its relation with organic nature, its empathy with all things, when the core of our breast moves from an animal to a mechanical imagination.
>
> —JAMES HILLMAN

That the heart is the primary organ of perception of the deeper aspects of the physical world around us was long recognized by ancient peoples. The Greeks had a particular word for it, *aisthesis*, from which our word *aesthetic* is derived.

Aisthesis describes a particular event, the moment when a human being encounters, and feels the impact of, the deeper soul essence in a thing of the physical world. The word literally means "to breathe in." The ancient Greeks knew that this moment of recognition was usually accompanied by a gasp, a breathing-in. Something from outside is entering into us, something with tremendous impact, something that causes an immediate inspiration, or breathing-in. It is important, and often overlooked, that at the same time the world is taking *us* in, we too are breathed-in. When we experience this sharing of soul essence, we have a direct experience that we are not alone in the world. We experience the truth that we live in a world of ensouled phenomena, companioned by many forms of intelligence and awareness, many of whom care enough for us to share this intimate exchange.

Aisthesis happens to us still, although few of us consciously understand what is happening. On seeing the Grand Canyon or coming unexpectedly upon a beautiful ancient tree in a forest, there is an immediate turning to the thing seen, a stopping, and then a gasp, a breathing-in, as the power of the thing is felt. But it doesn't happen often—not continually, as it has for much of our species throughout most of our time on Earth. For such soul sharing is impossible in a mechanistic universe that possesses no soul. The soul of a thing cannot leave it and enter us if it possesses no soul in the first place. Nor, if there is nothing there, can we be "inspired" by the breathing-in of the world.

Still, this basic experience—this aisthesis—has been at the root of human relationship with the world since our evolutionary expression out of the Earth. We are built to experience it, to be aware that each thing possesses a unique identity, its own particular *eachness*. We are made for the nature of each thing to pass into us through our hearts, which think about it, store memories about it, and engage in dialogue with it.

As with all developed human skills, it takes years of exploring and experimenting with the perceptual capacities of the heart for this perception to become sophisticated, just as it takes years to develop fluency with verbal language. Unfortunately, because we are trained out of using our hearts as perceptual, thinking organs during our lengthy school years, if we try to begin using this ability in later life, it is often a fumbling, awkward experience. Our heart intelligence is still working at a 6-year-old level, while our mind intelligence is absurdly further ahead.

Still, there is a great power in the world around us. It has not disappeared just because we no longer notice it. Fasting can help each of us reclaim personal perception of the sacredness within the world, within each particular thing. Spiritual fasting moves the faster from a rational orientation in a dead, mechanized universe to one in which the unique perceptions of the heart are noticed and strengthened—to a deep experience of the living soulfulness of the world. As the fast progresses, this process continues to deepen, and it strengthens our spiritual sensitivity and, in the process, helps us gain a deeper understanding of our own sacredness. During deep fasts there is often a period when the accumulated scar tissue that covers most of our hearts begins to be stripped away. This allows the heart to become flexible again, once more enabling us to use it as an organ of perception. This process is crucial, for it awakens in us, as Robert Bly has noted, a freshness that is inherent in the soul. (It is also no accident that on a strictly physical level, fasting is one of the most potent methods to heal long-standing heart disease.)

The freshness that Bly talks about is lost to many of us through years of living within an inanimate, dead universe. When

> Everything is speaking in spite of its apparent silence.
> —HAZRAT INAYAT KHAN

the world is redefined as dead matter, the physical forms of the world, once living places where soul resided, become mere cemetery markers where spirits once moved through the world. The grass in this new inanimate universe may be green and of a uniform cut, and (plastic) flowers may decorate the graves, but it is still very hard to live in such a cemetery. Once we accept that there is no soul in the world, that there is no living, intelligent, wise soul in ourselves, we collude with others in the breaking of our own spirits, and, literally, in the breaking of our own hearts. There is a reason that heart disease is the number-one killer of people in the Western world.

Experiencing the world as nonliving has powerful implications for how we live our lives. Our lack of real experience with our own soul, its intelligence and wisdom, and our failure to regularly engage the soul of the world and other living things cause all of us to live a half-life, cut off from the *luminous,* one of the primary sources of direction in life. The sense of alienation and depression that is so common now, the feeling that things have no meaning, the loss of a sense of personal direction in life, come directly from this misperception of the world. All too often these internalized experiences are also accompanied by a denigration of the physical world, a belief that it is less important than the spiritual. Sometimes this denigration even extends to a hatred of the body, often engendering a belief that it is a pollution of the spirit. This can force us up and away from the body and the material world when we seek the spiritual to enrich our lives. The emphasis shifts to transcending the body and matter itself—onward and upward rather than here and downward. As James Hillman comments,

> Western morality tends to put all better things up high and worse things down low. By this last century, growth became inexorably caught in this ascensionist fantasy. Darwin's thesis, *The Descent of Man,* became, in our

minds, the ascent of man. . . . By now the upward idea of
growth has become a biographical cliche. To be an adult
is to be a grown-up.[2]

New Age practitioners are often infected by this perspective
as well, and fasting is sometimes pursued in order to transcend the
physical, *not* to become more embodied, more whole, or more
holy in the physical. Our failure to recognize our uniqueness, that
we are here for a reason, that there are powers that care for us and
will help us in need, that there are ways to allow the deeper meanings of life to more fully enter our lives comes, to some extent,

> O human, see then the human being rightly: the human being
> has heaven and earth and the whole of creation in itself, and yet
> is a complete form, and in it everything is already present,
> though hidden.
>
> —HILDEGARD OF BINGEN

from a hidden denigration (even hatred) of ourselves, of the
body, and of our incarnation in physical form. Pre-Christian ori-
entations and even older Christianity did not make the same separation between matter and spirit—the location of the soul
someplace other than the world is a much later phenomenon. The
twelfth-century Christian mystic Hildegard of Bingen believed
profoundly in the holiness of the body and saw it as a reflection of
the patterns embedded within the cosmos. She insisted that as our
relationship with our soul grows, it "takes possession of the whole
body."[3] And only when the two are in harmony, with a deep and
abiding friendship, can the soul begin to touch the fabric of
heaven. To live in right relationship with Creation means honor-

ing the creation of the body itself, recognizing its inherent sacred nature, and developing a deep, trustworthy relationship with it. For there is only one place in all the Universe that has been made especially for you, and that is inside your own body.

We come into the world headfirst, diving out of the womb into the world. Our feet are the last things to emerge, and they remain the most difficult things to master. It takes some time for us to learn to stand on our feet, to be embodied in the world. Learning to be inside our own feet—planted firmly on the Earth—is one of the hardest things of all. The tendency to emphasize the head over the feet, the higher over the lower, remains a pervasive experience, one that is strongly supported by the belief that there is no soul or intelligence in inanimate matter.

Yet we are still surrounded by the livingness of the world, by its soul essence. As we live our lives, caught up in the day-to-day business of life, it is easy to forget who we wanted to be, to overlook the intimations we once felt of what we were to become, to dry up spiritually, and to lose a sense of our soul and purpose in life. The natural luminosity of the world, known to all children, fades, and we find ourselves, as we age, growing hungry for another kind of food. There is in each of us a hunger for our hearts to be touched by the livingness of the world, a hunger to feel the sacredness of life, a hunger for aisthesis.

It often takes a spiritual crisis to force us into a place where we begin to recognize this, before we begin to listen within. Yet it is only when we find our inner voice that we will also find our outer voice, that we will we begin to know what it is that we are really here to say.

One way to revitalize the self is to fast. And although this is sometimes used as a way to try and escape the body, it is also a means for truly coming to inhabit the body, to experience its sacredness and the particular soul essence that it possesses, to find not only holiness but also wholeness. For how can we be whole when inside ourselves we feel that there is something inherently wrong with our manifestation in the body? How can we be whole if we believe that there is something inferior about the physical form we have been given in this life? Matter and spirit, truly, are only two faces of the same thing. As Gandhi observed: "Just as there is an identity of spirit, so there is an identity of matter and in essence the two are inseparable. Spirit is matter rarefied to the utmost limit. Hence, whatever happens to one's body must affect the whole of matter and the whole of spirit."[4]

Historically, when human beings wanted to engage in deep fasting in order to recover or deepen their experience of the sacred, to find direction for life, they always went alone into wilderness, and they always fasted. For, as Hillman notes, "if we wish to find the responsive heart again we must go where it seems to be least present, into the desert."[5]

2

Spiritual Fasting and Detoxification

The World is the place of soul-making. —JOHN KEATS

He who buries his head deep into a nose-bag full of food cannot hope to see the invisible world.

—AL-GHAZZALI

There is a deeper self than the "I" that lives at the surface of our daily world. Each of us is born for a reason; there is a work we are here to do, some specific task that has been set before us. If we fail in the expression of this deeper self, if we do not find the work we are here to do, we find little in this life that can or will sustain us— physical food alone is insufficient for being satisfied, for being *filled* or feeling *full*. Given the nature of modern life, it is no wonder that the relationship between fasting, the sacred, and the reason for which we are born has been forgotten. For the truth that we are born for a reason, that there is something more to an individual life than going to school, getting a job, marrying, having children, having grandchildren, taking vacations, retiring, and dying has itself been forgotten. That the soul has its own destiny and that the life of the "I" that we know as ourselves is only a small reflection of that larger destiny is not taught in school and very rarely in churches of any religion. And if there is no memory, or teaching, in our culture that there is something special that our soul is here to do, that we live in the midst of the sacred, then the fact that there are processes that can help us remember that task and the sacredness of the world is also going to be forgotten, in fact, has been forgotten.

Fasting has always been viewed, in every culture that has existed prior to contemporary time, as an essential act at some time in every person's life for creating an opening in the self into which knowledge of the sacredness of the world and the work of the soul can come. Acts such as fasting, especially at the important transition periods of a human life—adolescence, middle age, old age, and death—have always been recognized as necessary. They open the self to direct experience of the sacred, to knowledge of the work that is here for the individual soul to do, and to the understanding of just what and who each of us is in this lifetime. This kind of knowledge is essential to living a fulfilled life. It allows the development, the nurturing, of a life grounded in deeper truths and oriented around essential meanings. It begins a process the ultimate goal of which is to completely and totally become who we are meant to be. Or, in Thomas Merton's words, "sanctity is nothing more than becoming ourselves."[1] This can never occur without discovering our calling.

This perspective, of course, is in direct contrast with contemporary perspectives about the nature of human life. All of us are infected to some extent with a certain belief about our lives—that we are only the product of a blending between our heredity and the environment in which we are raised, that we are in essence the victims of forces over which we do not have, and never have had, control. And while we do have free will within a certain range, in the most fundamental areas of life we do not. This is a discouraging view; it removes much of the beauty and joy from life—removes from it its mystery and depth—and is certainly inaccurate, though it is an inaccuracy that is often hard to see. Each day we are surrounded by shallow reflections, exhortations through the medium of television to follow the body's whims. Until, as Robert Bly notes, we believe "that the Montana hills were created to provide oil for central heating"[2] and that the way to self-fulfillment is the accumulation of more material goods—more clothes, more appliances, more food. This is a new phenomenon. Although this newer way of thinking has roots that go back to Aristotle, it only gathered its current tremendous force when Descartes's assertion that thinking was superior to feeling moved into the ascendancy in the seventeenth century. The crucial relationship of the soul to the body and of the body to the world began to be lost. We began to forget the truth of the soul's interior abundance. Now most people feel that to find the self, to develop the soul, one must dissociate from the physical world and break its bonds of connection to the body. Once it was understood that it was not in dissociation from the world that the truth of the soul's interior abundance would be found but in directly encountering it in its wildest state.

For as the poet Novalis says, "The seat of the soul is where the inner world and the outer world meet."

> Our work is to show that we have been breathed upon—to show it, give it out, sing it out, to live in the topside world what we have received through our sudden knowings from story, from body, from dreams and journeys of all sorts.
>
> —CLARISSA PINKOLA ESTES

The place where the inner and outer worlds meet has always been located, in all older cultures, in the same place: in wilderness. Each person who journeyed to the wilderness to seek intimations of their purpose did so in similar ways in all cultures on Earth in all times on all continents. They went carrying with them few material possessions; often they went naked; always they fasted.

In these older times, this journey into the wilderness (or sometimes a specific form of wilderness—the desert) was taken because it was understood that there is no place the sacred can more clearly be felt than in wilderness. And this work our soul is here to do is a work that comes from sacred realms, just as our soul is expressed into matter from sacred realms. In traveling to the wilderness, in leaving the cloth of civilization behind, in leaving the psychology of family and friends behind, in leaving food behind, the barrier between the sacred and the self thins and eventually dissipates. Knowledge begins to flow from the full into the empty.

And as the Buddhist teacher Joan Halifax remarks, "It is in these lonely places that the sacred mysteries, which infuse all, yet are visible to none, can find their way into the human mind."[3] "Nature's wilderness," she continues, "is the locus for the elicitation of the individual's inner wilderness, 'the great plain in the spirit,' and it is only here that the inner voices awaken into song. The inanimate sermon of pristine deserts, mountains, high plains, and forests instructs from a place beyond idea, concept, or construct."[4]

The decision to enter the wilderness and fast forces us into an immediacy of contact with the deeper aspects of ourselves and the

> To learn to see, to learn to hear, you must do this—go into the wilderness alone. For it is not I who can teach you the ways of the gods. Such things are learned only in solitude.
>
> —DON JOSE MATSUWA

interior world of those material forms that reside in wilderness. We begin encountering the world that our species was birthed into over long evolutionary time, the world that is deepest in our cellular memory. A door opens inside us, and something comes in from somewhere, some food that we need to be whole, to be holy. Often the return to wilderness or desert is accompanied by the decision to fast. This kind of fasting, spiritual fasting, is the intentional decision to encounter the hidden parts of the self and to find the hidden face of the sacred in everyday things. It is above all about becoming conscious of things you have put away and perhaps forgotten. It is about becoming aware.

Like many practices that are being rediscovered in the West, fasting is often stripped of its spiritual origins. Intentional fasting, historically, has usually occurred out of spiritual necessity. Spiritual fasting is often initiated or is necessary because of a stagnation in personal life—life seems confining, personal boundaries feel too small, the world is pressing in, and there seems to be no way out, no way into a more sustainable way of being. Spiritual fasting, especially in wilderness, allows the person to step out of a confining life by initiating an intentional encounter with death and suffering and, eventually, rebirth. It reconnects each person to the Universe around them and supplies new direction for life.

In the wilderness you encounter only yourself and the powers that exist and that have existed since before humans began, powers that reside in the Universe and the Earth. In this state, removed from the complexities that usually surround the self in daily life, the soul can begin to overtly work with its own renewal and detoxification. The inessentials drop away. Without these distractions, the barriers between the self and the Universe that enfold it begin to thin. As the Huichol initiate Prem Das describes it, "there is a doorway within our minds that usually remains hidden until the time of death. The Huichol word for it is *nierika*. *Nierika* is a cosmic portway or interface between so-called ordinary and nonordinary realities. It is a passageway and at the same time a barrier between two worlds."[5] Because fasting brings us so close to death, it also opens this doorway. Slowly, then ever more rapidly, as one fasts in the wilderness, the barrier between worlds thins

> All true wisdom is only to be learned far from the dwellings of men, out in the great solitudes.
>
> —IGJUGARJUK

and opens. The deeper meanings that are embedded in the world begin to penetrate the soul, and a food without which it is difficult to become human fills up and nurtures the self.

The recognition that human beings can make contact with the sacred by fasting and spending periods of time in isolation on the Earth is common throughout the world. In fact, the knowledge that humankind must periodically return to the wilderness or the desert for renewal is implicit or explicit in many of the world's religious traditions. It is common among all indigenous cultures.

Black Elk, the great Oglala Sioux holy man, noted there were many reasons to go into the wilderness to seek a vision, or "lament," as he called it. "But," he said, "perhaps the most important reason for 'lamenting' is that it helps us to realize our oneness with all things, to know that all things are our relatives; and then on behalf of all things we pray to *Wakan-Tanka* that he may give us knowledge of Him who is the source of all things, yet greater than all things."[6]

This remembrance of our oneness with all things, initiated by wilderness, is echoed in the Essene Gospel of John, wherein Jesus says:

> I tell you in very truth, Man is the Son of the Earthly Mother, and from her did the Son of Man receive his whole body, even as the body of the newborn babe is born of the womb of his mother. I tell you truly, you are one with the Earthly Mother; she is in you, and you in her. Of her you were born, and to her you shall return again. . . . For your breath is her breath; your blood her blood; your bone her bone; your flesh her flesh; your bowels her bowels; your eyes and ears, her eyes and ears.[7]

The Essenes were strong advocates of fasting in the wilderness, of bringing into the body the power of natural landscapes. "Seek the angel of fresh air," they insisted, "the angel of water, the angel of sunlight, and the angel of the earth, and invite them to stay with you throughout the fast."[8] Steven Foster and Meredith Little, in their book *The Book of the Vision Quest,* remind us of the importance of this reconnection with the holiness of the Earth, commenting that "the gift of love for our Great Mother is given to us at birth. But we often forget to remember. That is why it is sometimes necessary to go to her, to fast, and be alone with her, so that we can fully remember the kin relationship between our bone and her stone, our blood and her rivers, our flesh and the body of nature."[9]

This pattern of retreat to the natural world and engaging in fasting is common among indigenous cultures but also among Jews, Muslims, Hindus, Buddhists, Sufis, Taoists, and Christians. Some Christian orders, bearing in mind Jesus' 40 days in the wilderness, have historically endorsed the importance of wilderness retreat and fasting.

The Carmelite monk Father William McNamara comments that without periodic return to the desert, to wilderness, people can never know God. Time spent alone in wilderness allows human beings to stand back from their attachments to the things of the world and to recover connection to the basic elements of self and Earth, eventually finding the sacred center that is at the heart of all things. McNamara says:

It is man who needs the utter simplicity, the silence, and solitude, the emptiness of the desert. In the desert the difference between the essentials and nonessentials is reasserted; the distinction between the vital and moribund is rediscovered. The desert is a destruction of mediocrity which is compromise worked into a system. Mediocrity becomes impossible in the desert where everything is reduced to the rigid alternatives of life and death. Man then rises up out of a sluggish culture, regains a classical human stature as he responds to reality with authenticity and sensitivity according to a hierarchy of values in accord with the Supreme Value of ultimate reality.... Without the desert experience, man cannot achieve his destiny or fulfill his vocation.[10]

There are strong similarities between McNamara's perspective and that of Siya'ka, the Oglala Sioux who spoke with the ethnologist Francis Densmore in the early twentieth century.

All classes of people know that when human power fails they must look to a higher power for the fulfillment of their desires.... Some like to be quiet, and others want to do everything in public. Some like to go alone, away from the crowds, to meditate upon many things.... [One who decides to retreat to wilderness knows] it has long been his intention to make his request of Wakan'tanka, and he resolves to seek seclusion on the top of a butte or other high place. When at last he goes there he closes his eyes, and his mind is upon Wakan'tanka [the Great Spirit] and his work.... No man can succeed in life alone, and he can not get the help he wants from men.[11]

Black Elk notes that to receive the help each of us needs, we must go alone, fasting, into the wilderness, and truly ask for what we need. Anyone who does so, Black Elk says, "shall certainly be aided, for *Wakan-Tanka* always helps those who cry to him with a pure heart."[12] Often the touch of the sacred during such retreat brings knowledge of the work that we are here to do. Father McNamara writes that

if Christ needed to withdraw periodically into silence and
solitude, it seems egregious presumption to assume that
we can go on forever on our own steam with no direct
and intimate contact with the infinite Source of our being. . . . After St. Paul's dramatic conversion on the road
to Damascus, he immediately went straight to the Ara-
bian desert and spent a long time there. Obviously, the
full meaning of his vocation could not be penetrated unless he returned to the traditional source of spiritual
strength, the place where man meets God. Only after he
had steeled himself by prolonged retreat in the desert did
Paul plunge into his exhausting apostolic [work].[13]

The need to return to the place where the world-soul remains
strong, to touch the basic fabric of Creation, to strip away the su-
perficialities of daily life, to call on the sacred to help us in our suffering, to "lament," is universal. It is, further, an intentional act.
As McNamara says, "the experience begins with the free, deliber-
ate decision to suffer. It ends with the uproariously happy surprise
of being in harmony with the universe."[14]

> The soul breath of the fasting man's mouth is more fragrant be-
> fore God and better pleasing to Him than redolent musk.
>
> — MOHAMMED

Fasting is important during such retreats, and it is a very
ancient spiritual tradition. As the Muslim scholar Al-Ghazzali
notes, "the practice of fasting as a spiritual discipline is both ancient and widespread. It antedates Islam, even among the Arabs,
and from time immemorial has been observed in various ways by

Jews, Christians, and eastern and pagan religions."[15] Gautama Buddha set the pattern for retreat and fasting for those that follow Buddhism. In leaving his kingdom, Buddha shaved his head, left all earthly things behind, and went into the forest for six years, eating little, often fasting. He said that during fasting, "my soul becomes brighter, my spirit more alive in wisdom and truth."[16] Gandhi commented that fasting was an integral part of the Buddha's work: "When he saw darkness in front of him, at the back of him, and each side of him, [he] went out in the wilderness and remained there fasting and praying in search of light."[17] The Native American vision quest also involves a journey into wilderness accompanied by a minimum of four days of fasting. As the Anishinabe Betty Laverdure comments in the book *Wisdom's Daughters,*

> You go on the vision quest. You go with only one blanket. You stay in the winter. You don't eat or drink. . . . When you fast in this modern world, you have to separate yourself from the TV and radio. You have to rid yourself of the outside world. . . . Usually you just drink water or tea. You fast as long as it takes to put yourself at peace.[18]

Vickie Downey, a Tewa Pueblo native, comments in the same book that when we quest "we abstain from food, don't give anything to the physical. We have our body, then we have our spirit, and then we have our mind. [When we fast during a quest] those three things connect."[19]

Within Islamic tradition, fasting has long been considered essential to restoring strong relationship with the sacred, especially through its activation of the heart as an organ of spiritual perception. One of the followers of Mohammed asked him how to enter into a sacred life, and he replied, "Everything hath a gateway and

the gateway of heaven is fasting." Al-Ghazzali, the great Muslim
scholar, comments that "the main purpose of fasting is to purify
the heart and to concentrate all its attention on God." He who
comes to understand the real meaning of fasting "through the observation of his own heart . . . will not fail to find out where the
welfare of his heart lies."[20]

Among the Baha'i, fasting also has a long and continuing tradition. And within this spiritual tradition there has also been a
long-standing recognition of the importance of the heart to spiritual perception. "Fasting," one Baha'i text says, "is the cause of the
awakening man. The heart becomes tender and the spirituality of
man increases." It goes on to note that the

> material fast is an outer token of the spiritual fast; it is a
> symbol of self-restraint, the withholding of oneself from
> all appetites of the self, taking on the characteristics of the
> spirit, being carried away by the breathings of heaven and
> catching fire from the love of God.[21]

And among the Eastern Orthodox Church, where fasting for
Lent is still common, it is said that "we must open ourselves to the
love and strength that God offers freely. Fasting is a way of
achieving this openness. [Fasting does more than this, though, for]
on a cosmic level, the fast is [the] effort to put the world and life in
the world in its proper perspective."[22]

But perhaps the most famous practitioner of retreat and fasting in recent memory was the great Hindu/Jainist practitioner
Gandhi. Gandhi developed an exquisite sensitivity to the relationship between fasting and spirituality on many levels. By abstaining from food his palate became highly sensitized to the spiritual
food that fasting provides. He explored it as a science, examining

how his different attitudes and behaviors affected outcomes. He commented that "the mere fast of the body is nothing without the will behind it. It must be a genuine confession of the inner fast, an irrepressible longing to express truth and nothing but truth."[23] This is because "all fasting, if it is a spiritual act, is an intense prayer or a preparation for it. It is a yearning of the soul to merge in the divine essence."[24] Mohammed echoes this when he says: "Even if [a man] keeps his stomach empty he will not be able to remove the veil and see the invisible world unless he also empties his mind from everything except God."[25] For fasting to be successful, for such retreat to produce the outcomes desired, Gandhi observed that "fasting of the body has to be accompanied by fasting of *all* the senses."[26]

The deeper, spiritual elements of fasting are learned as we experiment with it, as we learn the territory. Islamic teachings, like those of Gandhi, make a distinction between superficial fasting and transformational, spiritual fasting. For, as Al-Ghazzali says, fasting, like "every act of worship, is possessed of an outward and an inner secret, an external husk and an internal pith. The husks are of different grades and each grade has different layers. It is for

> Fasting is a fiery weapon. It has its own science. No one, as far as I am aware, has a perfect knowledge of it.
>
> — GANDHI

you to choose whether to be content with the husk or join the company of the wise and learned."[27]

In going into the wilderness to fast, human beings encounter the true essentials of life; they strip from themselves the daily concerns that occupy so much of their time. Our daily concerns normally occupy so much time that we often begin to think they are all there is. As the religious writer Gloria Hutchinson comments, "ordinary life is a prudent shoplifter. While we are attending to other things, it depletes our inventory."[28] So this time away, in the original wildness of the world, allows us, for awhile, to walk away from the ordinary world and begin to focus on the deeper and more important truths of our souls.

Spiritual fasting in wilderness can be a deeply humbling experience. We travel without the accoutrements of civilization. We leave behind the shell of our daily lives—our homes, family, work, and tools. When we stop eating, we no longer receive sustenance in physical form but begin instead to rely on powers greater than ourselves and to seek a food only they can bring. We leave the physical food behind us and embrace a humility before the true food that is within all forms of creation—a food that we deeply desire. We enter a darkness, for we do not know what we will find when fasting and wilderness retreat begins. We initiate a journey into a dark place, a place in which our fears and hidden selves will come to the forefront of our minds and experiences. We enter a place with unique boundaries: the small area in which we experience the retreat, the few things we have brought with us, and the absence of food.

When we go into wilderness and fast, we journey because we feel we are in darkness, we journey because we have no sense of direction and feel lost. We fast because we have reached the limits of where we can go unaided. We desire to enter a new country of the spirit. We sense that there is something preventing us from entering therein. And we suffer.

Deep fasting always involves suffering. It is physically difficult. It is often undertaken because we are suffering in our daily lives and wish to heal ourselves. But on a deeper level fasting reminds us of the suffering that all of us inevitably encounter during our lives. It allows us to work with the nature of suffering itself, to understand it more deeply, and to connect the suffering inside us to a power greater than ourselves. Instead of continuing to avoid the deep need that our suffering indicates we have, we make the choice to turn and enter the darkness and intentionally engage it. Paradoxically, in such an act we find new life, new direction and joy.

Spiritual Detoxification

Deep fasting in wilderness also allows us to spiritually detoxify. The daily cares that occupy so much of our time, the demands of work, of social conventions, of family, and of things that we feel we "have" to do often accumulate, filling up our time, taking our attention, becoming toxins to the soul. The incessant mutter of the television, the continual sounds of technological civilization, the chatter that goes on continually in our heads—these things fill us up with distractions and take us away from who we are and who we knew we were to be when we began our journey through life. As our lives unfold, each of us is often channeled into paths that are not part of living a fulfilled life. Fasting and retreat in wilderness allows the inessentials of life to be stripped away, allows our souls to detoxify.

Like the physical changes that can occur during bodily detoxification, spiritual detoxification generates its own kind of alterations in the self. As the soul begins to detoxify, many things pass out of us, each leaving an image of itself in particular kinds of thoughts, feelings, and discomforts. These things are often concerned with *why* you are alive on this Earth and any childhood or cultural messages you have been given about that why. They concern your core beliefs about who and what you are, the capabilities you actually have, and those that you were taught you have. All of us have taken beliefs and spiritual attitudes into ourselves that are in conflict with who and what we are. These act as a kind of brake on what we can do with our lives and who we can become. We have accepted beliefs about the livingness of the world and whether or not we are cared for by powers much greater than ourselves. We have accepted beliefs and spiritual attitudes that continually reinforce a lessening of our spiritual stature—that keep us from realizing the work we are here to do and the unique destiny we have before us. As the fast progresses, these toxic beliefs and spiritual attitudes begin to flow out of the body. The important thing in such deep fasting is to allow yourself to empty, not only physically but also emotionally and spiritually. It is crucial to allow these beliefs and attitudes to flow out of you, to let them go, and in so doing to find what and who you really are. It is important to simply observe them, to allow them to flow out without doing anything about them. Cultivating an attitude of unattached watchfulness is helpful. Allow the fast to take you to its destination, simply observing what happens on the way. For, as Foster and Little comment,

> the fasting process is one of readying the soil for a seed to be planted in it. The seeker empties the body so that the spirit may be cleansed and filled. Abstinence from food encourages death, who wants to fill your emptiness. As you live naked, vulnerable, in alignment with death, your life is enhanced, made brilliant and terrifying. . . . You have nothing to put into your body but water. You cannot sit down with the evening paper and some munchies and

enjoy the view from the terrace. All you get is the view. And because you have nothing else to eat, you eat the view. You hear your empty belly gnawing on the silence. A cool breeze stimulates your taste buds; you salivate shamelessly. You feel your body turning inward upon itself for food, eating up your stores of glycogen and other sources of quick energy. The shadow of death nudges your heartbeat up and engenders a strange mixture of feelings: exhilaration and exhaustion. Your body is reduced to imitating the animal hunger that exists in the life around you.[29]

When you are empty, you are ready to be filled. And you cannot be filled with what you want unless what has been in your way is allowed to pass out. The shallow spiritual food that you have eaten each day for years has not nourished you as you wished and perhaps thought or were taught it would. The residual toxins, the side effects of shallow food, have to emerge from the deepest recesses of the self and exit. Some of these things as they pass out of you may be frightening, some difficult, many boring; some are surprisingly easy to let go of, and some are joyful. It is beneficial to attend to each step of the fast, to pay attention to what is happening inside you, and to work with it consciously. You are intentionally entering a new territory, intentionally deciding to suffer, to not eat. You are allowing yourself to empty so that something else, a better food, can fill you up.

Beyond all other things, the most important is to hold in the forefront of the mind the desire that you have. The desire for spiritual guidance and renewal, for the touch of the world-soul upon you, for light in the darkness. Merely considering a fast confronts each of us with a powerful journey of the soul. It signals to the deep self that the task before it is of a different order than those of daily life. This signaling initiates a movement toward the spiritual; it is the beginning of every fast. From the moment of this initial signaling, a request is being sent from the soul out to the sacred wildness of the world. Such requests are always heard, and the response depends on the clarity of the message, for the Universe will respond to whatever is uppermost in the mind, whatever is of most concern to the soul. It is this desire that will call to you what you need.

> The great sea has set me in motion
> set me adrift,
> moving me as the weed moves in a river.
> The arch of sky and the mightiness of storms
> have moved the spirit within me,
> till I am carried away
> trembling with joy.
>
> — UVAVNUK[30]

3

Emotional Fasting and Detoxification

We should eat enough good food to truly refresh ourselves so that there "be no lack of joy in our souls."

— HILDEGARD OF BINGEN

We eat the way we live. What we do with food, we do in our lives. Eating is a stage upon which we act out our beliefs about ourselves.

— GENEEN ROTH

The needs that motivate your decision to fast possess complex emotional elements. At the simplest, because food is so inextricably interwoven with our survival, our earliest memories of life and family, and so much a part of our families and cultural activities, the decision to abstain from food brings up a great many emotions. Fasting casts each of us into the choppy waters of our basic relationships with food. It initiates the release of emotional toxins that we have held on to, sometimes for years. These are most often unresolved family or cultural messages about food, love, self-worth, and survival.

As human beings, our earliest and most pervasive experience is touch—the touch of our mother's womb upon and around us and the feel of her arms holding us after birth. And it is one of the primary needs we have, to be held and touched and through that to experience the communication that we are loved, cared for, wanted. Our relationship with food is intimately interwoven with all of this.

Just after birth, exhausted from our long journey into the world, our umbilical cord is cut, and we are placed on our mother's chest, near the nipple. Soon we begin to seek nurturing there.

Humans at birth are helpless; our only tool for meeting our basic needs is the voice, our ability to cry. When we need the basic nurturance of food, we cry and are taken up to the breast to feed. From the beginning, how our mother responds to our cries for food, how she feeds us, and how she feels in giving us this most basic need are an essential part of our relationship with food. Whether or not it is okay for us to cry, to signal through the making of noise that we have an unmet need, is an essential communication that we absorb from the very beginning. The attitudes of the mother and father toward our helplessness and our needs are highly complex and multinuanced; nevertheless, they are communicated—we absorb them into ourselves—along with the food we are given.

All this shapes, at our deepest and most unconscious levels, our basic relationships with food. Like the foundation stones under a house, everything rests on these early experiences, and they subtly shape and alter everything that comes after. These early communications affect us throughout our lives. How our parents viewed our essential relationship with food as an essential nurturing substance becomes a lens through which we continue to see ourselves, food itself, and our relationships with others long after we have left home. At the most basic level, food is the thing that allows us to survive, and so how we relate to food is a reflection of how we view our own survival or our right to survive. Because it is so intimately connected to that other essential, touch, food remains tightly interwoven with concepts of touch and the basics of caring that are embedded in touch. Food, ultimately, holds within itself—because of all it means and has meant—the essence of touch, of caring, of nurturing, of survival itself. The decision to fast, to voluntarily refrain from receiving sustenance, brings to the forefront of consciousness *all* the associations we have with food, all the associations that we have been taking into ourselves from the moment of birth. For each of us, the associations are unique in their shape and form, for each of us have experienced a unique series of communications from our parents and our culture.

In many ways, relationship with food is the same for all of us. It is about trust and intimacy and survival. It is about trust because we have no choice but to trust our parents—we have no ability to provide the essentials for our own survival when we are infants. It is about intimacy because there is nothing more intimate than showing another our most vulnerable needs and asking for them to be met. It is about survival because, without this gift of food from someone so much more powerful than we are at birth, we cannot survive into adulthood. Thus food inevitably brings up issues of surrender, for if, after birth, we do not give in to the keeping of another the power over our life, we will not survive.

Fasting *always* brings up issues of trust and intimacy, survival and surrender. It brings up fears and thoughts and unresolved emotional complexes, sometimes those we might have thought long resolved. Fasting also brings up the cultural attitudes toward food that we absorbed as we grew, perhaps the belief that if we are thin we will be loved. It brings up the most basic beliefs we have about our bodies and what will happen to us if we change our bodily shapes. Fasting forces us into a confrontation with many of the darker parts of ourselves, deeper beliefs about ourselves and our worth as human beings, whether we deserve to survive, are lovable enough to deserve survival, whether our basic needs will be met. During fasting we confront all of our most basic fears about love, intimacy, surrender, and survival. And we often find that food is a cover under which we hide these most basic fears and beliefs. Intentionally refusing to eat pulls back the carpet and lets us see just what we have swept under it. And so fasting on an emotional level is, once again, a decision to become aware, a decision to not run from ourselves but to turn and face the darkness. When we do, the voices of those parts of ourselves that we have kept in darkness, suppressed by our behaviors with food, begin to take on strength and to grow in volume and start to be heard. Often, as the fast progresses, we find, suppressed under years of patterned behavior, the voice of our most vulnerable, infant self. The daily noises of life begin to recede, we enter a unique stillness of spirit, and then we start to hear, crying out, as it did after birth, our most vulnerable self, crying for a certain kind of sustenance that it needs but has never received. It cries out for food given in an atmosphere of trust and safety, where surrender is not defeat, where intimacy is acceptable, and survival a freely given gift from the powerful to the weak.

Fasting can be the beginning of changing our relationship

with food, with ourselves, and with others. It marks the beginning of learning to give to ourselves those things we never received in childhood. It prepares us, as Carol Normandi and Laurelee Roark so beautifully remark in their book *It's Not About Food,* for becoming our own best friend "so that we can perform the holy and sacred act of breaking bread with ourselves."[1]

Of Television and Babies

The American culture has an odd and not very functional relationship with food. *All* of us have been affected by it. How babies are fed in the United States and the pervasiveness of television are intimately bound up with this uniquely American dysfunction.

From approximately 1920 on, Americans stopped breastfeeding as a normal part of child rearing. This has had fundamental impacts on how we as Americans relate to food, how we feel about ourselves, and how we feel about others, love, intimacy, and getting our needs met. Instead of the continual touch that was evolutionarily a part of feeding in early infancy, there began to be, for many American children, little or none. For the immediate parental response to the cry of a hungry infant, Americans began to substitute the tyranny of feeding by the clock. Instead of the spontaneous flow of breast milk there was the substitution of synthetic formula. The outcome has been the emergence of eating disorders throughout the population and the creation of a nation of emotional ascetics—people who believe that deep needs should not be shown or, worse, met.

Television has been pervasive in American culture since the 1960s. From that time, most children have been raised with daily television as an emotional food staple. Many of the most pervasive commercials on television are those for food. These advertisements occur when the mind is most receptive to them and are invariably blended with images of people with a certain body type, age, and complexion. The lack of a healthy personal relationship with food since birth causes many people to be unable to tell just what kind of food will be satisfying to them. The images of the food that they do see, connected to the particular images that are most pervasive, lead people to impulse-buy food that will never produce the kinds of bodies they see in television commercials. These particular images of food inundate most of us throughout our lives, if we watch television, and contribute to considerable confusion about food and our relationship to it.

It is not surprising then that most Americans are overweight, are compulsive dieters, and associate body weight with the amount and kind of love they will receive. Twenty-five percent of all American men are dieting at any one time, as are 50 percent of American women. Our relationships with food, from the very beginning, are distorted and unhealthy. We, in reflection, have also become distorted and unhealthy.

These beliefs we have taken into ourselves about our bodies and the food we eat, about the physical world and our own physicality, can be extremely toxic. They are the emotional counterparts to the chemical toxins that our culture produces in the millions of tons each year; indeed, in many ways, they give rise to those chemical toxins in the first place. From our earliest years we have been taking in toxic communications, each of which has tremendous emotional weight, about our bodies and food. These are continually reinforced in the television shows and commercials we see each day, the communications of friends and families, and our own daily thoughts. Fasting not only allows the physical body to work through and release the chemical toxins that it has taken in but also allows our emotional body to release many of these emotional toxins.

When we consciously engage our deepest beliefs and fears about food and love through fasting, we begin to consciously examine the experiences we had in our earliest years, experiences that are closely connected to the beliefs we have about our worth, our right to be here, our right to receive nurturing. We begin to enter the territory of our most basic beliefs, to take them apart, to examine them, and to bring them into consciousness. We begin to understand our most basic relationship with ourselves, how we see ourselves, how we have long treated ourselves, how we do and don't use food. By raising all this to consciousness, we take the first step in *choosing* rather than accepting what we received when we had no choice. We begin to set ourselves free.

As Geneen Roth comments,

> Our relationship to food is a microcosm of all that we have learned about loving and being loved, about our self-worth. It is the stage upon which we reenact our childhood. If we were abused, we will abuse ourselves with food. The degree to which we are violent, abusive, self-punishing is in proportion to the degree of violence, abuse, and punishment we received. We learned how to do it by having it done to us.[2]

This is why fasting should be approached with consciousness and great delicacy. These questions must always be asked: "Is this fast an acting-out of unhealthy unconscious beliefs or an act of self-love? Does it carry on the unkindnesses of my childhood or assert my love of my self? Does it help me to become what and who I am to be or keep me as what I was?"

My Own Story

My own relationship with food is not an unusual one in the United States. I was born prematurely and spent several weeks in an Isolet—a crib where severely ill or premature babies were kept. At that time physicians did not allow babies in Isolets to be touched except very rarely by the nurses when performing medical or cleaning chores. Feeding occurred on a schedule that a doctor had predetermined. So I went from being surrounded by my mother's womb to complete isolation in which I was rarely touched, held, or loved. I had no contact with my family members, only strangers. No matter how much I cried, I was not held, nor was I fed. I came to believe that there was no relation between my asking for my needs to be met and them actually being met. My crying had nothing to do with being fed.

> Your body doesn't run on clocks. It doesn't know that breakfast is at eight, lunch is at twelve, and dinner is at seven.
>
> —CAROL NORMANDI AND LAURELEE ROARK

By the time I was brought home from the hospital I had become a "good" baby. I rarely cried, I continued to be bottle fed on a schedule, and my family, strongly American in their attitudes toward touch, rarely touched me at all. My mother was also a poor cook. There were a limited variety of meals we were regularly given, often on the same days each week.

There was tongue. One of the most frightening sights on coming home from school was finding a huge cow's tongue sitting in a pool of blood on the kitchen counter, seemingly ripped out of the living cow that morning. It was slightly curled, as if cut out in the middle of a scream. When served, it was generally over-cooked. It was heavy with too much cooking and emotional weight; I could rarely eat much of it.

There were also Benedictine sandwiches: cream cheese and chopped onions mixed together with green food coloring on white bread. There were stuffed green peppers: instant rice mixed with onions and high-fat hamburger and baked in a hollowed-out, usually bitter, green pepper shell, with a little ketchup and melted American cheese on top. There was canned fruit cocktail mix. I always ate the peaches and competed with my brother and sister for the cherry that gleamed up redly out of the bowl—an unlikely beacon of hope. There were frozen TV dinners, still a bit frozen in the middle. I still remember the horror of biting down into turkey the underside of which was laden with ice crystals.

I was 16 years old before I learned that the preparation and eating of food could be an entirely different experience. I had just left home and rented my first apartment when a friend, remark-ing in disgust on the canned corn I had served him, explained to me that it was much better with some butter and salt and pepper. I was 17 before I found out that pears are not grainy cubes in cans but when ripe from the tree one of the most marvelous fruits on Earth. I was 28 years old before I found out that the two-toned green thing I once ate as a child was an avocado.

Under stress I normally quit eating. When I did eat, I ate

poorly. I was a devotee of the monochrome theory of life. All my clothes were shades of brown. All my food was shades of brown. Then one day a woman who had taken a fancy to me (I am still not sure why, given my appearance and eating habits) treated me to a Sunday brunch. Confronted with really good food in inexhaustible quantity, I heaped full, and ate, plate after plate. I ate everything I took and went back for more and more and more. I felt a bit sick afterward.

The contrast between my poverty of sustenance and that moment of abundance changed everything. I decided that I would take myself out to eat every Sunday for a year; that I would do it in fact until at my deepest core I felt it was right and proper to receive an abundance of food.

The first emotional difficulty was the money. I had little, and spending it so lavishly brought up strong fears of survival. Every week I had to confront this fear of spending on myself. It took much more than a year to change that way of thinking.

The second problem was the food itself. My first inclination was to heap the plate high, and I felt that I had to eat *everything* I took. Even if it did not taste good to me, I would still eat it. I ate too many things I really did not like. I still remember the moment I realized that I could just take small amounts of anything that looked good and not eat it if I did not like it. I could simply go get another plate and get something I did like. From then on I would taste everything and then *only* eat those things I really enjoyed. In essence I was learning to give myself permission to discover what I liked and to eat as much of it as I wished. During this process I strove to, and finally succeeded in, turning off the parts of me that were continually engaging in criticism of what I was doing. Although it took a long time, eventually there came a time when I could completely, totally, and deeply receive the gift of the food that I was giving myself. I finally believed that there was enough food for me and that I would not starve. I finally reconnected my hunger with my eating—when that part of me cried, someone finally responded. And I could *choose*. I no longer had to take whatever came to me and eat it whether or not I liked it. I discovered hundreds of new foods. I discovered what I liked and what I did not.

I discovered as well that if I gave myself permission to eat whatever I wanted, I began to notice when I was full and not full, hungry and not hungry. The wisdom naturally inherent in my body, that is inherent in all our bodies, began to come forward again. I began to listen to what my body was telling me and found that it *knew* what food was good for me, what it wanted, and when it was full. It was very difficult to have no judgments about this process of learning, to simply observe what was happening, to find out what was true by exploring the territory without preconceptions.

I discovered, in time, that the small infant I had been was still alive within me and that I was not, that no human being is, a single personality. During this internal exploration of my self I found that all people are, in a certain way of thinking, born multiple personalities, that the infant, the four-year-old, the teenager, all of the people we once were are still alive inside us. When we live at home it is our parents' job to care for and respond to all these parts of ourselves. Our job as we age is to come to know ourselves, to make relationship with these parts of ourselves, to care for them, and to find peace with them. It is one of our most fundamental jobs as human beings to hear the voices of these parts of ourselves, to learn their needs, to meet them, to become our own best friend, our own parent. Only then, I later learned, can we be prepared to parent our own children. Otherwise our children only become opportunities for us to work out unresolved problems in ourselves, and the family parenting dynamics that we ourselves suffered from are passed once again into a new generation.

Fasting, eventually, became an essential element of my new relationship with food. But I was only ready to engage in fasting once I had really learned to eat, to receive sustenance, to engage in the holy communion of breaking bread with myself. I learned that giving myself permission to eat whatever I wanted was giving myself permission to have life. It was only when I had fully given myself this permission that fasting was not a deprivation or a replaying of my family-inherited relationship with food. Only then could I engage in fasting and not have it be an unkindness. Once I had given my deep selves the gift of being trustworthy enough for long enough so that they would surrender to me and receive nourishment from my hand, once I was reliable to them in this way, the decision to not eat was not a harmful act but a joint exploration into new territories of the self. It was not an abandonment of self but an embracing of new possibilities.

One essential truth about fasting is that if your underlying relationship with food is not conscious, fasting is often difficult. You cannot fast without challenging your most fundamental beliefs about food and nurturing. *If you believe that food is love, stopping eating will be experienced by your deepest self as a denial of love.* Food is always connected to love because of its close association with the initial nurturing we received and had to have to survive after birth. Because of how we were treated in our early years, many of us have a fundamental belief that we are not good enough, that there is something wrong with us, and that we are not worth loving. Fasting activates these core beliefs because it removes the cover for them—food.

Fasting is deciding to take the veil from our eyes, to become intimate with ourselves. It is a decision to encounter the pain from childhood that we have hidden underneath our relationship with food, to give the hungry part of ourselves a voice that cannot be

> We all have broken hearts. Every single one of us has had our heart broken at least once—in our families, from the loss or betrayal of a parent. Some had their hearts broken over and over again in terrible ways. When the heart of a child is broken, something inexpressible—and up to that moment whole and unquestioned—snaps. And nothing is ever the same. We spend the rest of our lives trying to minimize the hurt or pretend it didn't happen, trying to protect ourselves from its happening again, trying to get someone to love us the way we, as that child, needed to be loved. We spend the rest of our lives eating or drinking or smoking or working so that we never have to go back there again. Never have to feel the unbearable pain of our broken hearts.
>
> —GENEEN ROTH

ignored. Giving that part of ourselves a voice, we can hear it. Hearing it, we can respond to it. Responding to it, we become trust*worthy* to ourselves. We begin to find peace. If you are only using fasting to be thin so that you can be loved, it will not lead to the outcomes that are possible. It will, in the end, only continue a pattern begun long ago when you were very young.

Emotions and Fasting

The emotions we normally experience—though often unnamed— are far more complex than the simple ones of anger, sadness, fear, or joy. The touch of the external world upon us expresses itself in highly complex and sophisticated feelings. These thousands of subtle feelings are the language of our hearts. That language is as sophisticated and as comprehensive as the language of our minds, the language we know as words. Unfortunately, some time between the ages of four and six we are trained to quit developing the language of our hearts. Reclaiming our body wisdom means becoming sensitive to the touch of the world upon us, beginning to be aware of the thousands of emotional complexes that that touching generates, and beginning to decipher the meaning of those emotional complexes. These emotional complexes are communications to us about the deeper meanings we encounter in the world as we go about our daily lives. They are communications to us about what we need as well. They are messages from the wisdom of our body about what it needs, about what the many parts of us need, about what we, as whole complex living beings, need in order to remain whole and healthy and ourselves. During fasting, the sensitivity of the body to the world around it increases substantially. Subtle perceptions long hidden under food, television, and daily life begin to be noticed again. The touch of the world upon us, communicated through the scores of sophisticated emotions that our bodies generate, begins to be felt more strongly each day the fast progresses.

The denial of the complex feelings that exist within us as a birthright of our humanness often causes us a loss of connection between the soul essence inside us and the soul essence outside us. For the subtle feelings we have are also communications to us from the soul of the world; they continually tell us that we are not alone. And embedded within those feeling-communications is information from the world about the things we need—including just what kinds of food—in order to be whole.

But in addition to these complex feeling-communications from the world around us, fasting also stimulates the more basic feelings of fear, anger, grief, and joy.

Our culture constantly teaches us, and all new generations, that feelings are untrustworthy. In addition, the only feelings that are consistently culturally supported are happy ones. We are rarely supported in letting go and letting ourselves drift down into the feelings that lie below the surface of our social selves. We are rarely encouraged to become explorers of our own psyche, to ready ourselves for the most daring exploration of all, that of the inner world in which we live. Fasting opens the doorway to this exploration of the psyche. The feelings that we uncover in such explorations are *all* important ones. They all exist for a reason. They all possess wisdom and meanings that we need in order to become ourselves. Only in giving up the cultural prohibition of having "bad" feelings can we find out just what those feelings contain.

This is important because as soon as anyone starts to fast, or to even consider a 'fast—unless they have done it many times— many uncomfortable feelings and thoughts often arise. One of the most immediate is "Will I survive?" Death is an inevitable confrontation with which the self has to grapple when the decision to fast is made. Fasting is more than anything an engagement with personal mortality and the rebirth that follows such an engagement. When we decide to fast we decide to examine our own relationship with survival, and this means directly encountering death. These are heady topics, and one reason that fasting should be undertaken with consciousness and deep thought. In any engagement with our own death we have the opportunity to deeply examine our lives, to explore what we have done and not done, and to decide what we wish to do in the future. We have the opportunity to revise or alter the path we have taken, to make new choices, to begin anew.

Remember:

Anger is energy to solve a problem. It often signals that there has been an infringement of our essential nature.

Fear is a signal that there has been some change in circumstances that directly affects our survival.

Sadness is letting go of something.

Joy is the natural response to healthy functioning of our living selves.

Because of the nature of fasting and the emotional confrontations it generates, fear almost always arises. It is exceptionally important that the surroundings for fasting be supportive and nurturing so that the parts of you that are frightened can feel as comforted and nurtured as possible. They have to feel that you have not abandoned them. It is, of course, possible to force yourself through a fast in spite of feelings of fear—to "John Wayne" the process. But you risk simply reinforcing the messages received in early childhood. A much better approach is to consciously work with the fear, to examine its roots, to see from where inside you it arises, and to seek to understand the underlying meanings that are attached to it. In this way it is possible to directly respond to the fear so that the need it represents is met. Fasting is an essential act of learning to really hear, and respond to, the self.

Anger, too, is an essential emotional component of fasting. There are few difficult things in life that we do not need anger to help resolve. Anger, more than anything, is energy to solve problems. It is a source of soul force, an impetus to move through obstacles, and it is most efficiently channeled if this is realized and the anger consciously used in each moment it arises. What is the source of the anger? Is there something under it? What is it, exactly, that you want, that will alleviate the anger? Is there a particular part of you that is angry, and if so, what does it want? And more to the point, what can you do with the anger to help you make it through the problem you are facing?

Grief is, as well, nearly always a part of fasting. During a fast each one of us inevitably encounters not only the unkindnesses that we have done to others but the unkindnesses we have done to ourselves. Especially poignant are the necessary and healthy hungers

> If you were sexually abused at the age of five, told no one, and began eating compulsively, you will be left with the raw terror that you felt at five when, at age forty-six you stop using food to comfort yourself. Unless you do something with the terror or sadness or rage, with the feelings of abandonment or engulfment, with messages you received and internalized about your self-worth and lovableness, unless you bring them to the surface where you can look at them, turn them over and decide if and where they belong now, they stay rooted in the childhood soil in which they were planted . . . feelings do not go away just because they have no relevance to our present situations. Like shadows that disappear when you face them, feelings disappear when you name them, and only then.
>
> — GENEEN ROTH

in ourselves that we have not met, the hungers for love, for caring, for touch, for true intimacy, for a work that is meaningful, for a life filled with the soul's abundance and with soulful interchange with the world. The feelings of grief that arise are most effectively dealt with if they are treated much like those of fear—examining what they are, where they come from in the self, and what important meanings are concealed within them.

But grieving takes time. Geneen Roth comments that "many people want to fly past grief into forgiveness because grief is so uncomfortable and forgiveness so sweet."[3] The time necessary to grieve is one of the most important gifts we can give ourselves. It is only through the taking of time to grieve that we also give ourselves the gift of the new self that is coming into being on the other side. It is an essential part of becoming whole, becoming holy, becoming ourselves. If we fake our emotional state in the mistaken belief that false niceness and forgiveness make us a better person, we do not become a better person but only a caricature of a human being. Underneath it all are the original feelings still crying out to be heard and received. Encountering our most basic beliefs when we intentionally change our relationship with food means having the courage to enter a new territory of the self and actively find out just what it does mean to become authentic and real and ourselves.

This cultural imperative to feel only good feelings at all cost is indeed carried out at great cost. We try to suppress the deepest communications from our hearts and deeper selves; failing that, many of us turn to pharmaceuticals, whose only purpose is to apply tremendous chemical leverage to suppress just those feelings that our culture says we must not feel. Continually trying to look on the bright side interferes with our finding the wisdom that lies in the fruitful darkness. Continually striving upward toward the light means we never grow downward into our own feet, never become firmly rooted on the Earth, never explore the darkness within and around us, a darkness without whose existence the light would have no meaning. To become rooted in ourselves, in the world, we have to grow down as much as we grow up. To find the fertilizer that feeds our growth, we need the rich dark loam that lies within our deepest selves.

When the parts of you that have been locked up so long are first allowed a voice, allowed out of the small room in which they have been imprisoned, they will possess a tremendous amount of energy and force. They have been storing up their rage and need for a long time, often decades. They can often seem frightening, the amount of energy they have stored within them immense. It takes a lot of work to make peace with them, to come to terms with them, to hear their cries and decipher the underlying need. It takes a lot of work to meet that need. The process can be frightening and exhausting; the rewards are great. For what you are doing is an ecological reclamation of the self.

During fasting it is important to keep a journal and allow these parts of yourself a voice in its pages. It is important to have a safe and supportive space for fasting so that you have the place to hear these voices and allow them to speak. It is important that you not judge the parts of you that come forward during fasting. Just observe them, hear what they have to say, and come to know them. They are a great source of energy and power, and they have a powerful effect on your life, whether you know it or not. Their needs will not go away just because you repress them or do not listen—quite the reverse. Fasting is not easy; it is mining the deepest realms of the self, and it is often hard work. But the reward is great.

One of the most difficult things about fasting is encountering hidden beliefs about food and nurturing. Too often a primary motivation for fasting is the purification of the self in one form or another. This is problematic because the decision to purify is often based on the assumption that there is something wrong with how

> Many people can listen to their cat more intelligently than they can listen to their own despised body. Because they attend to their pet in a cherishing way, it returns their love. Their body, however, may have to let out an earth-shattering scream in order to be heard at all.
>
> —MARION WOODMAN

you are. That perhaps you are too filled with fat, or impure, or sick, or unclean, or unwholesome, or bad and that only a grim and intense purification will alter your body enough so that you will find love. Fasting is, in these instances, sometimes used so that the person fasting will be "okay," be thin enough, filled with enough Light, be *clean* enough to finally be loved by another human being or even by God.

All of us have been given many messages that we are unclean or are somehow impure or "spoiled." That deep core belief manifests itself in lineages of fasting that are concerned with "getting the unclean out of us." This can lead to a number of oppressions of the body during fasting, including various forms of bowel cleansing such as enemas and colonics. This is not to say that those processes may not sometimes be useful, but often the underlying reason for their use during fasting or "cleansing" fasts is to try to remove uncleanness from the body, to try to remove the stain that so many people believe lies on them so that they can become pure enough to be loved and so that the feelings of shame—about themselves and their bodies—that they carry will dissipate and bother them no more.

This, in the final analysis, is only a form of violence to the self and a perpetuation of the unhealthy beliefs of childhood and of our culture. It is a form of self-hatred. It comes because what was mirrored back to us as we grew was not love of who we are and of our bodies but its opposite. We can decide to not perpetuate these old beliefs at any time. The price of freedom is encountering the parts of ourselves we have put away and denigrated, learning to love them, hear their voice, and respond to their needs, and never abandoning them again.

When you fast you come face-to-face with the fragmented and split-off parts of yourself that you have not acknowledged. The willingness to stop defending yourself against the pain you once felt, and the pain that comes from this fragmentation, is essential.

You may find, as well, when you begin to fast, that a voice listing all your limitations and failures begins chattering in your head. It may turn out that the continual eating of food is what stops this voice during your daily life. Now that you are fasting, there is nothing to stop the sound it makes.

What is "under" the inner critic? To find out, when you hear that voice in your head that tells you that you are not good enough or beautiful enough or lovable enough, stop. Turn and look at it. Just be patient and wait and keep looking. What is its shape? Does it have a face? Whose? Slowly work with it, send your questing self into it, and look for what is there. Underneath it there is something else. Underneath that first face there is another one. In me it is a part of my self that is afraid that I will not be lovable, will not receive the nurturing I need to survive, if I act differently from the way my parents wanted me to, if I move and crawl and cry and smile and laugh and make noise and shout out the things I need. If I in any way stand out and am not monochrome. If I am alive. It took many years for me to reassure that part of me that I would not abandon myself, that *I* would make sure that those things it needed to survive would be provided, and that I would never stop listening to what it was asking of me. When it finally believed me, after a very long time, it began to relax and smile and laugh. It became one of my strongest allies. One of the most effective early stages of making good relationship with this part of you is simply to watch it—to become a nonjudgmental observer, to become aware. How often does this part of you tell you these kinds of things about yourself? How much does it affect your actions and choices? Do you like how it feels?

You might notice that you turn to food if there is some problem bothering you. If you have not gotten enough attention from others, enough strokes, you might find yourself eating instead. What do you use food to cover up in your life? What meaning does food have to you? What does it represent? Is it hard for you to eat in front of people? Do you reward yourself with food? What feelings do you associate with junk food? With healthy food? What thoughts do you have about your body? What part of your body do you like most? Least? Fasting can begin bringing up your deepest thought patterns about your body and your relationship with food. During a fast you can start to become aware of how much time you spend thinking about and preparing food. Thoughts of food can become constant during a fast. Once you begin changing your deepest relationships with food, you enter unknown territory. This new world must be learned one step at a time. The shape of its terrain will be unique to your needs; you must find it by being intimate with yourself. If you become aware of your deeper relationship to food, you will begin to discover not only what your physical hungers are but your emotional and spiritual hungers. Each of us has different ones. Only you, by coming to deeply know yourself, can determine what each of them is for you.

Paying attention to the subtle cues of your body is essential. One of the primary things that happens during a fast is the reestablishment of a sophisticated relationship with your body. By stepping back from your immersion in the world of television, work, food, and social interactions, you give yourself the space to focus on your needs, what is going on internally with you and you alone, and what your needs actually are. It gives you the space and time to slow down and really attend to yourself. What your body needs and doesn't need can be seen much more clearly. These needs, these communications from your body, are often very subtle. The immersion in the demands of the world distracts the mind from the subtle emotional, physical, and spiritual communications from the deeper self. Stopping that immersion allows you to attend to those communications, to discover their shape

> How do you begin to seek the wisdom of the body? You do it one step at a time—eating experience by eating experience. Every mealtime is another chance to feed yourself in a natural way, to take care of yourself as you have never done before, to love and trust yourself to answer your own call. This way of self-care moves out into all other areas of your life, but it starts with the precious act of feeding yourself meal by meal, day by day.
>
> —CAROL NORMANDI AND LAURELEE ROARK

and how they manifest themselves, to interpret just exactly what they mean, and then to meet them.

Thus one of the most important teachings of fasting is learning to be present in the body. Because most of us have been taught to denigrate our bodies, we have learned to dissociate from the body, to view it simply as a kind of car, albeit an organic one, with no intelligence, wisdom, or soul.

We have been trained to believe that others, *experts*, know more about what our body needs to be healthy than we ourselves do. Reclaiming health means reclaiming the livingness of our body; it means coming to our senses again, learning to reinhabit the physical form we have been given, and listening to our own body's wisdom, its communications to us about itself and its communications to us about the world in which we live—especially this includes its intelligent communications about the food we take into our body. The body actually has highly sophisticated mechanisms for analyzing food—for determining just what food it wants to eat, how much of it, and when. Fasting reconnects us to this sensitivity of the body and initiates a relationship with food that is new and fresh and marvelous. When we begin to trust the internal wisdom of our body, that trust is repaid to us a million-fold. That trust, percolating through the deepest layers of who we are, will affect every part of our lives.

When you begin to change your relationship with food by deciding to fast, you are also changing deep and often unconscious agreements you have about food with your family. Remember, they are not the ones who decided to change, you are. Thus you are breaking an agreement, albeit an unconscious one. They are likely to be upset with you even if they cannot say exactly why. The best thing to do is to discuss the matter with them out loud, without blame, and ask for support. If they do not give it, and you want to proceed anyway, tell them you have to do it for yourself, apologize, and then go ahead if you are still determined to do so. Make sure that you arrange your fasting in such a way that those old agreements cannot become activated—for example, by fasting at home with an uncooperative family.

Once you start to fast, your fast will bring up in your family and friends all of *their* unresolved issues about food. The voice inside them that tells them things about food will take over their mouths and begin to speak to *you*. Your actions in choosing to fast can be a tremendous confrontation of their deepest feelings and fears about food and being loved and safe. It is important to take this into account when you decide to fast.

One of the most important reasons to remove yourself from your normal surroundings when you fast is so that you can step outside of the cultural messages we all receive daily about the body, its shape, its worth, and the food we (should) put into it. Many of these messages reinforce earlier messages we received as children about ourselves and our food, and this makes it all the harder to fast without such a separation.

During deep, retreat fasts, you are removing yourself as well from the many emotional foods you receive daily from family, friends, and coworkers. An added aspect of fasting can simply be a sort of emotional fasting—the abstinence from daily emotional foods. These can be as simple as the look a loved one gives you in the morning when you rise, the camaraderie that flows between coworkers, the daily sharing that happens between friends. The abstinence from these regular emotional interactions during retreat fasting brings up the needs these emotional foods meet. Such abstinence allows these needs to rise to consciousness and to be examined. It is often the case that a number of the emotional interactions that each of us have daily also contain within them certain kinds of emotional toxins—unkindnesses that, while having tremendous impact, are normally overlooked. Many of these emotional toxins have their roots in our initial family relationships—we simply find new people to continue these old messages after leaving home. Deep, retreat fasting allows the toxins embedded in unhealthy emotional communications to flow out of the self. The clarity of mind that comes from fasting can be applied to these kinds of emotional foods, and just as with physical food, the *kinds* of emotional food you take in when you return from your fast can be changed to kinds that are more healthy and nurturing and less filled with toxic messages about who you are, what you are, and whether or not you deserve to be cherished and loved for who and what you are.

4

Physical Fasting and Detoxification

If we live in a world whose soul is sick, then the organ which daily encounters this sick world-soul first and directly through aisthesis will also suffer as will the circulatory channels which transmit perceptions to the heart.

—JAMES HILLMAN

The truth is that your body, every ounce of fat you carry, is not your enemy. It is a part of you, a part that has been shamed in a culture obsessed with thinness.

—CAROL NORMANDI AND LAURELEE ROARK

A great many amazing things happen in the body during fasting. The body, as I have said, has its own wisdom—and it knows a lot about fasting. We are evolutionarily designed to fast, and the body knows how to do it very well.

Fasting allows the body to rest, to detoxify, and to heal. During this time, the body moves into the same kind of detoxification cycle that it normally enters during sleep. It uses its energy during a fast not for digesting food but for cleansing the body of accumulated toxins and healing any parts of it that are ill. As a fast progresses, the body consumes everything it can that is not essential to bodily functioning. This includes bacteria, viruses, fibroid tumors, waste products in the blood, any buildup around the joints, and stored fat. The result is that the body eliminates its toxin accumulation, just as during a fast the emotional and spiritual bodies eliminate theirs. And although fasting has always been concerned with both spiritual and emotional healing, it has, as well, been recognized for millennia as one of the most powerful forms of healing for the body.

The physical dynamics that occur during fasting are complex, and to understand them it helps to understand the process that your body goes through while fasting. The information on physiological changes that are discussed in this chapter, however, primarily pertains to water fasts. Juice fasting initiates similar but milder changes; the movement into ketosis, for example, is only partial during a juice fast. This is discussed in more detail later in the chapter.

Detoxification of the Body During Fasting

Heavy toxin loads can poison any ecosystem in which they accumulate. It does not matter whether this is the physical body or the closed environmental system we call the Earth. Because the body is a microcosm of the Earth itself, the toxins that are produced each year as a byproduct of technology damage our internal ecology just as they damage the Earth. Clarissa Pinkola Estes echoes this thought when she comments: "The body is like an Earth. It is a land unto itself. It is as vulnerable to overbuilding, being carved into pieces, cut off, overmined, and shorn of its power as any landscape."[1] Because we live in a time in which the physical world is so disrespected, it is nearly impossible for any of us to not absorb attitudes and perspectives that cause us to treat our bodies as things and to deliver to them the same kind of ecological disruption that we, as a species, are visiting on the Earth.

All of us are historically unique in that most of us have developed in a constant bath of synthetic chemicals. This is a unique evolutionary event—we are, in fact, guinea pigs in a vast uncontrolled experiment. This puts unusual strains on us and our bodies that are unique in evolutionary history. All of our bodies must somehow find a way to detoxify not only the toxins that humans have encountered throughout their evolutionary development but also these historically unique synthetic chemicals. In general, fasting enhances the body's ability to detoxify toxins—even these

> Last year each of us, on average, swallowed three pounds of flavorings, colorings, preservatives, glazes, antispattering agents, emulsifiers, bleaches, and other additives with our food.
>
> —JOAN MORGAN, M.D.

unique synthetic compounds—and regenerate any tissues that have been damaged.

There are four primary sources of toxins that people are usually exposed to: (1) airborne pollution that we breathe in or absorb through our skin, (2) pollutants we ingest on or in our foods,

(3) pharmaceuticals, and (4) toxins from bacteria and viruses, including those normally in our intestinal tract.

Airborne pollution can be paint fumes, the vapor from gasoline that we inhale when we fill our gas tanks, smokestack pollution, internal combustion engine gasses from cars and trucks that are present in tiny amounts in the atmosphere, or even synthetic perfumes, deodorants, and hairsprays. Some of it, like spilled gasoline, paint thinners, perfumes, and deodorants, can also be absorbed through the skin.

Pollutants that are in or on our foods include such things as synthetic fertilizers, pesticides, growth hormones, and so on that are sprayed on, planted with, injected into, or fed to our plant and animal foods.

Pharmaceuticals are a major source of toxins that people ingest, sometimes daily for many years. These substances are not evolutionarily natural to the human body. That is, the human species has not encountered these particular chemical structures during its long evolutionary history and has no experience in how to deal with them. When making pharmaceuticals, companies often attach synthetic molecular segments to natural substances such as testosterone in order to make them assimilate more quickly, to make them more powerful, or even to make them longer lasting. These unique molecules are not recognizable by the body as anything that it has encountered in its long evolutionary history and so are detached from the natural molecule. They must then be excreted, deactivated, destructured, or stored. It has often been the case that these unique molecular segments cause problems years later. Cancer is one common outcome in athletes who have used synthetically altered testosterone.

The bacteria and viruses that we encounter each day are another source of toxins. Normally they are efficiently handled by the body. If we do become ill, however, these organisms can sometimes release toxins into our systems. Often these toxins are in fact the reason we feel ill. The bubonic plague bacterium, for example, does not actually cause illness itself; rather, the disease comes from the toxins that it releases into the body as it dies. This is why killing all the plague bacteria in the body with antibiotics will sometimes produce death if there are too many of them. Another more common source of bacterial toxins are the bacteria in our intestines. They produce a great many chemicals as they engage in their own life cycles, and all of these are released into our intestines. Some of these chemicals are essential to our health (such as vitamin B-12), and in fact, if the bacteria that live in our bowels are killed off, we cannot survive. Some of the chemicals they release, however, can have toxic side effects if our bodies are not working well. The impacts of bacterial toxins are often much more severe or enhanced in those who have taken antibiotics or have eaten a predominantly Western diet of refined foods. The historical diet eaten by human beings throughout their long evolutionary history normally has contained hundreds, sometimes thousands, of local ecosystem plants. Such plants are high in potent plant chemicals that play essential roles in deactivating the toxins that human beings encounter during their lifetime. The reliance on a highly refined diet has removed these potent plant compounds from our diets, and one result is a more powerful negative impact from intestinal bacterial toxins.

All these toxins affect health by disturbing healthy cell function. Detoxification processes such as fasting allow the body to focus not only on restoring healthy organ function but also on attending to the needs of individual cells. Fasting rests the immune system, the detoxification systems of the body, and the entire digestive system. Instead of these systems analyzing, breaking down, and transporting the thousands of chemicals coming into us from our diets or dealing with the chemicals that come into us from our daily immersion in a technological culture, fasting allows them to rest, retreat, recuperate. Refraining from eating allows the body, just as it allows the spiritual and emotional body, to step back from its constant immersion in life and readjust its relationship with itself, the substances it has taken inside itself over the years, and the environment in which it lives. Deep fasting puts the body into a state that is normally only experienced during sleep, one in which the liver and other detoxification systems can focus exclusively on detoxification, repair, and regeneration.

Each human body is a microcosm of the Earth itself. The wounds so easy to see in the world around us—the clear-cutting of the rain forests, the ecological devastation in so many ecosystems—are only a larger version of the ecological devastation in our own bodies, much of which comes from the same kinds of sources. The first act of ecological reclamation of the world is the reclamation of your own body. The human body is evolutionarily adapted, just as is the Earth, to respond to damage and the buildup of toxins within it. Wetlands are one primary system the Earth uses to cleanse itself of toxins. One corresponding organ system within us is the liver. The liver's cytochrome P450 enzyme system is a unique system that is highly stimulated by fasting; its focus is the removal, deactivation, or reuse of toxic substances within the body.

Cells, the basic unit of the human body, need three primary things: food, communication with other cells, and a clean and healthy environment within and around themselves. Cells utilize some fifty different nutrients as food. As a cell eats these nutrients and produces energy, it is working hard and accumulates a lot of "sweat," or biochemical waste products, that must be eliminated every day. Cells, just like people, don't like to sit and stew in their own wastes. Their waste products are removed through the blood and lymphatic systems. Those deposited in the blood are taken to the liver and kidneys for handling. There they are either converted into other more useful substances or are eliminated from the body. They are usually eliminated through feces, urine, sweat, and respiration. When toxins build up faster than they can be eliminated, cell health is disrupted, and the initial stages of many chronic diseases begin. This kind of condition has been known in Eastern healing traditions for thousands of years. It is called *poisoned blood,* which refers to the presence of an overwhelming toxic burden that the body is unable to handle.

Cells contain a number of important organs that can be affected by toxins: DNA, mitochondria, and the cellular membrane. Each cell also lives within an extracellular matrix whose health is crucial. All of these can become damaged from toxin overload.

Actually *not* a software program, DNA is more accurately described as a highly flexible organ of the cell; DNA is not fixed but is very mobile and in many instances can rearrange its structure. The DNA strand in each cell is highly sensitive to toxins, especially synthetic petrochemicals. The DNA constantly degrades and is repaired by the cell; however, when toxic loads rise so high that the cell or body cannot deal with them effectively, the DNA in cells can begin to experience so much damage, so often, that it cannot be repaired.

Mitochondria are formerly free-living bacteria that have been incorporated within many types of living cells. They oxidize, or burn, ATP (adenosine triphosphate) in the presence of oxygen to produce the energy that cells need to live and function. Mitochondria also possess DNA strands, and although they were formerly thought irrelevant, DNA strands can also become damaged by toxic overload, thus affecting mitochondrial health. While the DNA in the nuclei of cells is protected by detoxification enzymes that break down toxic chemicals and heavy metals, mitochondrial DNA and other organs appear to be much more susceptible. When they begin to malfunction, there is a significant drop in the body's overall energy levels. Large disruptions in their functioning can lead to more serious conditions such as chronic fatigue syndrome.

The cellular membrane, created from special fatty acids, serves as a barrier between the cell, other cells, and the extracellular matrix. It is studded with receptors that can be thought of as communication ports. These receptors analyze anything that touches the cell and decide whether or not to open a gate in the cellular membrane to let substances into or out of the interior of the cell. When the cells can no longer detoxify themselves or are experiencing a heavy toxic load, toxins can begin binding themselves to the fatty cellular membrane and its receptors. This begins to interfere with a cell's ability to perceive the communications it should and with the passage of material into and out of the cell. This makes it harder for the cell to transfer waste products out and nutrients in. An additional complication is that once a cell wall has toxins attached, the cell is altered enough that the body's immune system can sometimes begin to attack it—the beginnings of some types of autoimmune diseases.

The extracellular matrix in which cells are embedded is a living substance, not merely an inert medium that holds the cell. It is made up of collagens and polysaccharides that form a water-filled gel. This matrix controls blood supply to the cells. If the matrix loses its consistency and thickens, the flow of nutrients into the

The Physiological Changes of Fasting

Many of the most dramatic changes that occur in the body during fasting take place on the first three days of the fast. These occur as the body switches from one fuel source to another. Normally, the primary form of energy that the body uses is glucose, a type of sugar. Most of this is extracted or converted from the food we eat. Throughout the day, the liver stores excess sugar in a special form called glycogen that it can call on as energy levels fall between meals. There is enough of this sugar source for 8–12 hours of energy, and usually it is completely exhausted within the first 24 hours of fasting. (Once the body shifts over to ketosis or fat as fuel, this new fuel is used to restore the body's glycogen reserves.) Once the liver's stores of glycogen are gone, the body begins to shift over to what is called ketosis, or ketone production—the use of fatty acids as fuel instead of glucose. This shift generally begins on the second day of fasting and is completed by the third. In this interim period there is no glucose available and energy from fat conversion is insufficient, but the body still needs fuel. So it accesses glucose from two sources. It first converts glycerol, available in the body's fat stores, to glucose, but this is still insufficient. So it makes the rest of what it needs by catabolizing, or breaking down, the amino acids in muscle tissue, using them in the liver for gluconeogenesis, or the making of glucose. Between 60 and 84 grams of protein are used on this second day: 2–3 ounces of muscle tissue. By the third day, ketone production is sufficient to provide nearly all the energy the body needs, and the body's protein begins to be strongly conserved. The body still needs a tiny amount of glucose for some functions, however, so a very small amount of protein, 18–24 grams, is still catabolized to supply it—from ½ to 1 ounce of muscle tissue per day. Over a 30-day water fast, a person generally loses a maximum of 1–2 pounds of muscle mass. This conservation of the body's protein is an evolutionary development that exists to protect muscle tissue and vital organs from damage during periods of insufficient food availability.

From the third day onward, the rate of the breakdown of fatty acids from adipose (or fat) tissue continues to increase, hitting its peak on the tenth day. This 7-day period, after the body has completely shifted over to ketosis, is where the maximum breakdown of fat tissue occurs. As part of protein conservation, the body also begins seeking out all non–body protein sources of fuel: nonessential cellular masses such as fibroid tumors and degenerative tissues, bacteria, viruses, or any other compounds in the body that can be used for fuel. This is part of the reason that fasting produces the kind of health effects it does. In addition, during this period of heightened ketosis the body is in a state similar to that of sleep—a rest and detoxification cycle. It begins to focus on the removal of toxins and the healing and regeneration of damaged tissues and organs.

Ketosis

One of the major physical changes that occurs during fasting, ketosis takes place only when the intake of carbohydrates (the source of most of the body's glucose) falls far enough to force the body to use fat stores for fuel. Normally, as soon as carbohydrates are consumed and detected by the body, the pancreas secretes and releases insulin. This is used to help process the glucose that the body gains from carbohydrates. Ketosis can occur only when insulin levels fall nearly to zero, and they will only do so if no car-

bohydrates or sugars are being ingested. Insulin in the blood inhibits the release of fatty acids from adipose tissue. This is an evolutionary conservation tactic—in periods of abundant food, the
tendency for the body to increase fat stores is maximized. These
fat stores are saved until they are needed during periods of low
food availability.

So when carbohydrate intake falls nearly to zero for longer
than 24 hours, the liver's production of a chemical called glucagon
rises. This activates an enzyme in adipose tissue called lipase,
which starts the process of lipolysis, or the conversion of fats to us-
able ketones. Glucagon's ketogenic and lipolytic actions are inac-
tivated by even tiny amounts of insulin; this is why during fasting,
in order to maximize ketosis, no carbohydrate intake should occur. As a fast progresses and as ketone concentration in the blood
remains higher than glucose, the body begins to prefer ketones or
fatty acids to glucose as a source of energy.

The first stage of ketone production is the conversion of fat
triglycerides into fatty acids and glycerol. These triglycerides are
initially formed by the body from the chemical reworking of fatty
acids, acetyl CoA, and glycerol. During fasting, the body reverses
this conversion process, changing triglycerides into fatty acids,
acetyl CoA, and glycerol. The glycerol is used to make sugar,
from which the body gains about 16 grams of sugar a day, and the
acetyl CoA is used to make ketones—acetoacetic acid, acetone,
and beta-hydroxybutyric acid. The heart and, as fasting progresses, the brain use these ketones for energy. The fatty acids are
transported through the blood to the liver; this is why during fasting, fat levels in the blood, including cholesterol, rise.

Once lipolysis, or fat conversion, is initiated, the body's first
step in using fatty acid tissues for fuel is breaking them apart into
smaller molecules. Most fatty acids are long molecular chains of

carbon atoms, 16 or 18 carbon atoms long. The body breaks these apart, successively taking off carbon chains that are 2 atoms long. They are a form of acetic acid—the same kind of acid we call vinegar. These 2-atom-long carbon chains are used to form acetyl CoA and ATP. The major form of energy used by the mitochondria (the energy producers) of cells is ATP, which is usually formed from glucose. Still, the body can also make ATP from fatty acids, ketones, and certain amino acids.

As the body begins using fat stores and breaking them down for use, they are removed in reverse order: the most recent fat stores are used first, and so on. As these fat stores are broken down, the chemical toxins within the fats are released. Each of these different toxins will have different effects on how you feel. (In addition, the associated emotions or reasons you accumulated that particular fat will also be released.)

During fasting, when the body is ingesting insufficient amounts of carbohydrates from which to make glucose, acetyl CoA is taken to the liver, which turns it into acetoacetic acid, acetone, and beta-hydroxybutyric acid. The liver then sends this acetoacetic acid into the blood for transport to the rest of the body for use as fuel. During this period large amounts of ketones are secreted into the blood. The heart, brain, and muscles are all able to use this semidigested form of fat as fuel, much as they usually use glucose, though the brain tends to prefer beta-hydroxybutyric acid. As the fast progresses, the liver begins to focus more and more on the production of ketones, and the renal cortex of the kidneys begins to focus on the production of most of the daily requirements of glucose.

The presence of so many acidic ketones in the blood begins to tilt the delicate pH of the body toward the acidic side. The body works to correct this through several mechanisms, mostly by the conversion of bicarbonate into CO_2 (carbon dioxide), which is exhaled. When this buffering capacity is exceeded, the body begins excreting ketones in the urine, and some acetone may also be excreted through respiration, leading to an odd taste in the mouth—metallic or chemical is how most people describe it. Some people use special urine testers that are made to detect the presence of ketones in the urine to determine just how completely their body is in ketosis.

Testing for Ketosis

You can buy urine testers that are used to find out if your body is in ketosis. One of the better known is Ketostix; another is Keto-diastix.

During this shift from glucose to ketone bodies as fuel, the entire body, including the brain, has to get used to a different fuel. All bodily functioning is affected, just as a car is affected by using a different kind of gas. Over time, the body and brain become accustomed to a certain type of fuel, and you become used to how they work on that fuel, so much so that *how* you feel and function on that fuel never rises to conscious awareness. During the fast, as the body uses up its habituated fuel and begins shifting to alternative systems, the normally unnoticed physical, mental, and emotional effects of your fuel begin to rise to conscious awareness. One particular aspect of this is an alteration in brain function; there is an adjustment phase in mental functioning during a fast as the brain shifts from one fuel to another.

The first part of this alteration occurs on the second day of the fast, the interim period when there is no longer sufficient glucose for normal mental functioning. As sugar stores fall and the body is denied carbohydrates during the initial stages of the fast, the brain's supply of sugar drops. This leads to lightheadedness, sometimes dizziness, and difficulty in complex problem solving. On the third day, when the body has shifted over to ketosis as a primary source of fuel, the brain begins to have enough fuel but it is a different fuel. How you feel and how your brain works on that fuel are markedly different. This is not because the fuel is inferior to glucose—the body can use either fuel with great efficiency. The difference is felt because it has been so long since you and your brain have used this fuel to function. It is more an outgrowth of habituation to glucose than anything else. During this period, the mind is often a bit fuzzy, thinking clouded. The brain, and you, will get used to beta-hydroxybutyric acid as a primary fuel source over the 3–7 days it takes for ketosis to reach its peak. When in full ketosis, the mind simply works somewhat differently. Thinking can be just as acute, but it tends to be slower, more reflective, more studied and deeper, and—aside from thoughts of food or ending the fast—less inclined to dwell on future plans.

Again, the slight difference in mental functioning that is experienced from ketones is an evolutionary development of exceptionally long standing. The human body is evolutionarily designed to use both glucose and ketone bodies for energy; there is nothing inherently better about either of them. In fact, ketones are the first fuel we use. Immediately after birth all babies are in a constant state of ketosis because they are living on the high-fat diet of mother's milk. Because the baby is receiving no carbohydrate calories, the baby's body begins life with ketosis as its primary method of producing energy. It is only the switch to solid foods that begins the alternate energy cycle based on glucose. Some researchers' findings indicate that ketone bodies, because they are the body's first fuel, may actually be the body's preferred fuel. Studies have shown that they stimulate the heart, adrenal cortex, skeletal musculature, and the brain to better functioning than glucose. The brain's periodic utilization of this alternative fuel during periods of food shortages (or fasting) also seems to have long-term beneficial effects on brain and central nervous system function. Electroencephalograph (EEG) data and endocrine testing generally show significant improvements after fasting.

Again, glucose, while it is the predominant fuel source for most of us, is only a later fuel, the outcome of eating solid food. Breastfeeding, throughout the history of our species on this planet, normally extended for 24 to 60 months, and it produces primarily a ketosis-based metabolism. This type of metabolism is evolutionarily intended to be our first type of metabolism, and certain physical developments can only occur when ketosis is taking place. It is not an abnormal type of metabolism, simply unremembered for most of us. Evolutionarily this ability of the body to utilize ketones so effectively as fuel is extremely useful. Excess food is stored as fat during bountiful times; then during lean times the body can switch back to a ketosis-based metabolism and use fat reserves for energy. The body is highly adapted to periods of low food availability and, in response, as the biochemist and professor Maria Linder comments,

> reduces its need for protein-dependent [glucose production] by boosting its production of ketones, a fuel *alternative* to glucose for *most cells*. Circulating ketones reach maximum levels after about ten days of fasting and now substitute for much of the glucose requirement of the central nervous system. This drastically reduces the need for catabolism of muscle protein.[2]

The body is evolutionarily designed to protect its muscle tissue (of which many major organs, most notably the heart, are composed) from deterioration during long fasts by having an equal ability to utilize ketones for fuel during long periods of reduced food availability.

Ketosis versus Ketoacidosis

Occasionally some concern is raised by a few medical practitioners about the body's being put into ketosis by fasting. Often there is a confusion between ketosis and ketoacidosis. The two are somewhat similar processes but at root very different in nature. Ketoacidosis occurs when concentrations of ketones rise very high in the body because of abnormal physical states. It most commonly occurs among some Type I diabetics and alcoholics. *Fasting does not cause ketoacidosis.* Ketosis occurs when ketone bodies in the blood rise above normal blood ketone levels (0.2 mmol/l) yet remain below the extremely high levels that are associated with ketoacidosis. Ketosis is a normal part of the body's functioning; ketoacidosis is not. The body normally possesses natural biochemical mechanisms to regulate the level of ketosis that occurs in the body, how long ketosis lasts, and what happens when it is occurring. These protective mechanisms are not functioning in Type I diabetics and alcoholics.

The kidneys' analysis of the contents of the blood during filtration plays an important role as one of these protective mechanisms. Sensing high ketone acids in the blood, the kidneys excrete ammonia to balance the acid/base levels in the body, thus preventing ketoacidosis. This regulation by the kidneys also protects the body from the loss of large quantities of sodium and potassium ions in urine during fasting, something that can occur during ketoacidosis. Only on the second day of fasting, prior to the complete shift to ketone production, does the body excrete significant amounts of sodium and potassium in the urine. This stops once healthy ketosis is in place. The conservation of sodium and potassium ions helps maintain the body's electrolyte balance and its overall healthy functioning during fasting.

Ketosis versus Starvation

There is also sometimes a confusion about the difference between starvation and fasting. Occasionally some people confuse ketosis with starvation. They are very different things.

There is a lot of fat loss during fasts—one of the reasons why so many people choose to fast for health reasons. Fat provides 3,500 calories of energy per pound—it is, in fact, the most efficient storage of energy in the human body. One gram of fat provides 9 calories of energy, compared to only 4 from 1 gram of carbohydrate or protein. It takes a *lot* of exercise to lose a pound of fat. Fasting, in contrast to exercise, uses up fat extremely rapidly by converting it to ketones for use as fuel. People generally lose 1–2 pounds per day of a fast. The more fat your body has, the more is converted to fuel each day.

Starvation, on the other hand, is the use of the body's protein, which is held primarily in muscles and organs, for fuel. This only occurs after *all* the reserves of fat and all other excess tissues and molecules stored in the body—bacteria, viruses, fibroid tumors, stored pollutants, and so on—have been exhausted. Once all other fuel sources are consumed, the body begins to use its own essential proteins for fuel. This is starvation. The majority of people—even very thin people—have enough reserves to fast a minimum of 45 days, and usually much longer, without their bodies beginning to utilize essential protein reserves. As a water fast progresses, the desire for food drops to nearly zero. It will rise again, sharply, when the body has used up all its available fuel reserves and is at the point of needing to use proteins for fuel. This usually occurs somewhere between 45 and 120 days into a fast—though fasts of much longer duration have been done. Those that have experienced it report that the tremendous hunger that occurs at this time cannot be mistaken. It is generally considered to be the primary indicator that it is time to break a very long fast.

Once the body has fully entered ketosis, it begins to work on healing itself. The range of conditions that have been shown to respond to deep fasting are remarkable.

Serum Leptin, the Obese Gene, and Weight Loss

Extended fasting, meaning anything longer than three days—the length of time it takes for ketosis to fully initiate—produces a number of interesting changes in the body. As is not the case with dieting, during fasting the body completely shifts over to an entirely different fuel source. The cessation of carbohydrate intake and the shift to ketones causes a great many alterations in physiological functioning that never occur on diets. An important one is that the body's food thermostat is turned off for a while and then is reset at a new and lower setting. After prolonged fasting, the body tends to prefer fats, which it rapidly oxidizes rather than stores, and to dislike carbohydrates, especially starches. There is a corresponding drop in glucose tolerance, which is to say that it doesn't take much sugar to satisfy the desire. The end result is that less food is desired, and the weight loss that occurs during fasting tends to be conserved.

The body will eventually desire higher food intake, but this takes time, much longer than with dieting; the changes associated with fasting tend to last for a long time. Studies of severely obese people who participated in extended fasts have found that it takes between 2 and 7 years for them to regain their prefast weight if they do not change any of the environmental, emotional, and spiritual factors that originally led to their weight gain. Fasting seems to be something that needs to recur regularly as part of a lifestyle choice, at least once per year or every other year. Evolutionarily, it seems necessary to experience on a regular basis for us to maintain health.

At the same time that weight loss is occurring, fasting significantly increases sensitivity to what foods are desired, are needed, and feel good in the body. This seems to occur in part from a heightened awareness of the perceptions of the vomeronasal organ (VNO).

This organ is something possessed by all mammals on Earth; it is located above the palate and behind the nose. It has one function: the identification of the substances we are taking into our bodies. Molecules from whatever we breathe or taste are separated from our food or air and taken to the VNO and attached to receptors there. These receptors connect directly to the brain, to a part of the brain whose function it is to analyze the molecules. Physiology and behavior shift, sometimes significantly, in response to what the brain determines about the molecules. For example, it is widely known that women who live together will eventually all menstruate at the same time of the month. A researcher, intrigued by this phenomenon, took the sweat of a volunteer, diluted it one part per million in distilled water, and applied it to the upper lip of other women scattered about the town. Within a few months they all started menstruating at the same time of the month. The body initiated highly specific physiological changes based on only one part per million of the substance that was secreted in the first woman's sweat.

As we go through our daily lives we become less and less sensitized to the information our brain culls from the VNO. After fasting, however, the body is highly sensitized to everything the VNO perceives. Smells take on an exquisite layering and can be perceived as compositions of multiple chemicals with great depth. This heightened sensitivity extends to *how* the body responds to the food it is offered. Fasting allows you to develop a new and deeper relationship with your body; your body will begin telling you what foods it likes, what foods are good for it, what foods it needs, and what foods it wants through the subtle communications that exist between the brain, the VNO, and your conscious awareness. In general, for a long time after fasting, your body will rarely want starches, lots of heavy meats, or sugars.

The body will also significantly change how it works with a number of important substances that it produces. Among them is *leptin,* a particular substance that is produced by the so-called obese gene (that has been much in the news the last few years) in its interactions with the body. Leptin levels positively correlate with obesity and seem to play an essential role in the body's storage and conversion of carbohydrates into fat tissue. Pharmaceutical companies are engaging in a considerable amount of research to find substances that can reduce leptin levels in the body as a way to initiate weight loss. Fasting, however, has significant impacts on leptin levels in the body. Obese gene expression of leptin is decreased by fasting; in fact, levels fall fourfold during water fasting. More important, serum leptin production does not rise to its previous levels after the fast is broken. The body's circadian rhythm of leptin activity itself is not affected by fasting, only its baseline levels and the height of daily peaks. Production patterns remain the same, but the amount of leptin production falls and remains low during and after fasting. Another way to say this is that the body's fat storage thermostat is lowered and reset at a lower level once eating resumes. Once the obese gene lowers its production of leptin, serum leptin levels fall extremely low. Not surprisingly, this directly reduces the transport of leptin into the brain. By the third day of fasting, as ketosis is initiated, leptin production falls to the low that it will maintain throughout the fast; it will not rise again until the fast ends.

Leptin has been found to have a regulatory impact on hormonal synthesis and secretion within the growth hormone releasing factor (GRF)–human growth hormone (HGH)–insulin-like growth factor-1 (IGF-1) axis. As leptin levels begin to fall in moderately overweight people, from the first to the third day of fasting this causes the beginning of an increase in HGH secretion and IGF-1 production. This keeps levels of free fatty acids and their rate of oxidation high during fasting.

And while women generally tend to have higher levels of leptin, possibly an evolutionary adaptation to ensure that the childbearers can more optimally survive food shortages, fasting abolishes sex-related differences in leptin secretion. It falls to zero for both sexes during fasting, but after fasting, women do not generally have higher levels of leptin than men. The disparity only begins to recur over time.

While fasting and exercise training both cause similar drops in leptin levels, ketosis is not completely initiated during exercise, and the levels of fat usage are much lower.

Fasting, Human Growth Hormone, and IGF-1

Human growth hormone (HGH), produced in the pituitary gland in the center of the brain, is converted in the liver to other growth factors such as insulin-like growth factor-1 and -2 (IGF-1 and -2). Human growth hormone is short-lived in the body, and the liver converts it to IGF-1 as a more stable compound that can be transported throughout the body in the blood. (To *keep* it stable, it is bound to a very stable protein, IGF-1 binding protein, or IGFBP.) Fasting stimulates a more than twofold increase in IGF-1 binding protein. Levels rise from an average of 30ng/ml to 340 ng/ml during fasting. The particular IGF binding protein produced during fasting is also much more potent than the one that is normally present in the body.

Human growth hormone has a number of important effects in the body. It stimulates muscle formation, increases lean tissue development, stimulates fat loss, and increases tissue repair, and it enhances brain function, bone strength, energy levels, metabolism, tissue growth, cell replacement, sexual function, organ health and integrity, and enzyme production. Many of its functions act to reverse the numerous impacts of aging. Human growth hormone reaches its peak production in adolescence and normally declines from about age 30 onward. It is reduced 25 percent by age 40, 45 percent by age 50, and 60 percent by age 60. The pituitary gland is always capable of producing as much HGH as ever, but in later life it needs initiating factors such as fasting to do so.

Insulin-like growth factor-1 also has a number of important effects on physiology. It stimulates osteoblast formation and activity, chondrocyte formation and activity, and collagen formation.

Osteoblasts are responsible for the formation of new bone, and increased IGF-1 levels have been shown to directly contribute to new bone matrix formation. Because more bone is usually lost later in life than is produced, bones become weakened and breakage is common. Increasing IGF-1 levels through fasting directly contributes to the alleviation of porous bone: osteoporosis.

Chondrocytes, on the other hand, are the cells involved in the formation of cartilage. This higher activity is possibly why most arthritis conditions tend to self-repair during fasting.

Both HGH and IGF-1 also act to maintain protein conservation in the body during fasting, when HGH acts to strongly inhibit the body's ability to break down muscle tissue protein. As HGH levels rise, glucagon and free fatty acid (FFA) levels also increase, and HGH acts to stimulate the oxidation of FFAs by the body as its primary fuel source.

Severely obese people need to fast longer before they begin to show significant HGH increases; 10–14 days can sometimes be necessary. Obesity, perhaps from the suppression of HGH by continually elevated leptin levels, causes the body to act much like those of people with hypopituitary (HGH-deficient) problems.

HGH deficiency causes a variety of problems that the severely obese also experience: increased body fat, high blood pressure, and high cholesterol levels; and decreased muscle tissue, cardiac output, energy, immune function, libido, skin elasticity, wound-healing rate, mental function, memory, strength, and bone mass and density.

Fasting and Diabetes

When carbohydrate intake ceases during fasting, the body's production of insulin slows and eventually stops. Corresponding decreases occur in serum glucose, C-peptide, and proinsulin. Insulin is initially synthesized as proinsulin. C-peptide is a polypeptide that remains in the bloodstream when proinsulin is converted to insulin. Although insulin levels fall during fasting as leptin levels decrease, the body's cellular sensitivity to insulin rises—which is one of the reasons fasting has been found effective for treating Type II diabetes. While there is plenty of insulin in the bodies of people who have Type II diabetes (not so for Type I), the body's cells are unable to respond to it effectively—they have become desensitized to it. This alone makes fasting important in Type II diabetes. A second reason is, of course, that Type II diabetes is often initiated by weight gain in adult life. Fasting corrects both conditions.

The beta-cells, located in the pancreas, are the source of insulin secretion in the body. Research has found that the beta-cells contain leptin receptors which monitor the amount of leptin in the body—the beta-cells alter their production of insulin in response. Insulin is secreted by the beta-cells in response to the intake of sugar or carbohydrates—the insulin helps cells take in glucose and facilitates the cellular mitochondria in using it to produce energy. Prolonged high levels of insulin increase the serum levels of leptin, which in turn causes more fat storage and greater weight gain. The increase in the serum levels of free fatty acids during fasting stimulates beta-cell electrical activity, which is partly responsible for the alteration in beta-cell enzyme and polypeptide production. Fasting seems to act as a potent tonic for pancreatic function and cellular health. It has been found to be the most efficient method of reversing Type II diabetes.

Cholesterol Levels and High Blood Pressure

Cholesterol and triglyceride levels in the blood tend to rise during fasting, even more so in those with cardiovascular disease (though by the end of the fast they tend to drop much lower than they were prior to the fast and remain low afterward). It might seem odd that cholesterol levels rise during a fast, since there is no food intake; however, the body's use of adipose tissue for fuel releases fats into the bloodstream for transport to the liver for processing. This is one source of higher cholesterol levels. But another and perhaps more significant source of increased cholesterol in the blood is the body's breakdown of atheromas during fasting. Essentially, this means the cleaning out of arterial plaque and the transport of the removed fatty cholesterol back to the liver for use as fuel during ketosis.

In general, the increase of cholesterol deposits in blood vessels in those with cardiovascular disease is due not to increased cholesterol intake in food but rather is a symptom of the body's repair mechanism for damaged blood vessels. As blood vessels wear out over time, and because of the constant exposure of the vessel linings to the oxygen in the blood, tiny cracks eventually appear in the inner lining, or endothelial tissue, of the vessel walls. Among other things, oxygen in the blood causes an oxidation to the vessel linings, and over time the vessels begin to look much like a garden hose that has been left too long in the sun. They begin to lose their flexibility, and when they are bent, small cracks appear. The body, in an attempt to repair the damage, coats them with cholesterol. When the cracks heal, the cholesterol is removed and transported through the body for use elsewhere. Cholesterol is an essential element of our health; to give only one example of its importance, all steroid hormones—like male androgen, testosterone, and the female estrogen estradiol—are made from cholesterol.

During cardiovascular disease the body is often unable to heal the vessels, due to toxic overload, and can only cover the cracks with cholesterol—a temporary, Band-Aid approach, not a complete repair. During extended deep fasting, the body can begin the actual work of repairing these cracks in the blood vessels. As the fast progresses, serum levels of vitamin E and beta-carotene increase, and they are transported through the blood for use in helping to repair the damaged endothelial lining of the blood vessels. Studies have shown that, during fasting, endothelial tissue heals significantly and its activity normalizes, *especially* in those with cardiovascular disease. The cholesterol that was being used as a patch is then released back into the blood for use elsewhere. Deep fasting, because it actually repairs the cracks in the blood vessels, produces lower serum cholesterol levels once fasting is completed. These levels tend to remain low unless vessel damage recurs.

Because endothelial cell activity normalizes, endothelial-mediated vasodilation increases. This causes a lowering of blood pressure. (Because blood pressure lowers, the extremities often become cold during a fast, and you may feel very dizzy upon standing suddenly, so don't stand suddenly.) Water fasting produces significant reductions in mean arterial pressure, heart rate, and oxygen consumption. Cardiovascular activity tends to normalize, especially in cardiovascular disease, and to remain normal long after the fast. As only one example, in one clinical trial of hypertension and fasting, 174 people with hypertension were prefasted for 2–3 days by eating only fruits and vegetables. They then participated in a 10- to 11-day water-only fast, followed by 6–7 days postfast during which they ate only a low-fat, low-sodium vegan diet. Initial blood pressure in the participants was either in excess of 140 mm of mercury (HG) systolic or 90 diastolic or both. Ninety percent of the participants achieved blood pressure lower than 140/90 by the end of the trial. The higher their initial blood pressure, the more their readings dropped. The average drop for all participants was 37/13. Those with stage 3 hypertension (over 180/110) had an average reduction of 60/17. All those who were taking blood pressure medication prior to fasting were able to discontinue it. Fasting has been shown in a number of trials like this one to be one of the most effective methods for lowering blood pressure and normalizing cardiovascular function. Blood pressure tends to remain low in all those using fasting for cardiovascular disease once fasting is completed.

During fasting the heart lowers its production of glucose-handling proteins and increases (up to 50 percent) its production of those proteins involved in fatty acid transport and metabolism. Part of the tendency of cardiovascular values to normalize is due to the movement by the heart to better metabolize FFAs and to its movement away from glucose. The sugar that is transported in blood, itself, can cause severe damage to blood vessels over time. Part of the reason that Type I diabetics experience so much cardiovascular disease is that their constant high blood sugar levels corrode the blood vessels. Dropping the levels of sugar in the blood allows the body to focus on healing without having to deal with the corrosive effects of sugar at the same time.

Other Physiological Changes During Fasting

Throughout the first three days of a fast, there is also an increase in the levels of epinephrine, norepinephrine, and cortisol. During the first two and a half days of a fast, cortisol production doubles. And while high cortisol levels can normally produce a number of negative side effects, these effects are actually reversed during fasting. How the body works with its powerful hormones alters considerably during fasting in order for a healthy homeostasis to be maintained.

Researchers have noted that "human beings evince strong adaptive homeostasis both monohormonally and bihormonally to fasting."[3] Individual hormone production and hormone interactions are evolutionarily structured to change in the event of fasting. These hormonal increases and alterations tend to stimulate a higher burn rate of FFAs during fasting, help conserve muscle tissue, and help maintain body homeostasis.

As FFAs are released into the bloodstream, the plasma abundance of a unique protein called fasting-induced adipose factor (FIAF) also rises. FIAF is present throughout the body but most heavily in adipose, or fat, tissue. It appears to have specific endocrine functions, acting as a hormone throughout the body. Not well understood, FIAF appears to play an essential role in the regulation of energy homeostasis during fasting. Peroxisome proliferator activated receptor alpha (PPAR) also increases during fasting; it stimulates the production of compounds necessary for fatty acid metabolism during fasting.

Skin tone is often affected during lengthy fasting of 14–45 days, especially in younger fasters. When you are fasting, the levels of several extracellular matrix components of the skin, such as glycosaminoglycans (GAG), decrease. There is also a corresponding decrease in the body's synthesis of these macromolecules. Lactate concentration in the skin, which occurs naturally in the aged, doubles during fasting; lactate naturally inhibits GAG biosynthesis. Fasting also inhibits collagen synthesis and increases the amount of IGF-1 binding proteins in the skin. There is a significant decrease in skin collagen content, collagen biosynthesis, and prolidase activity during fasting. What all this means is that extended fasts often can produce a very aged-looking skin, especially in young fasters. The condition disappears when the fast is broken. Oddly, this process seems to be remarkably beneficial for the skin once the fast is broken, though no one knows why. After fasting the skin generally takes on a much more youthful appearance and possesses better regeneration capacity, tone, and luster.

Thyroid hormone levels (except T4) generally decrease during fasting. Thyroxine (T4) levels tend to normalize if they have been low or to remain the same during a fast. An essential hormone in maintaining many of the body's metabolic processes and functions, T4 facilitates cell production and maintains normal cellular growth, stimulates more efficient oxidation in the mitochondria, facilitates the repair and regeneration of damaged or diseased tissues in the body, and helps maintain healthy heartbeat and brain function. Healthy T4 production is also essential in successful weight loss for those who are obese. The thyroid gland helps regulate how fast or slow the body's metabolism is by the amounts of T4 it produces. Too much T4 and it races, too little and it struggles sluggishly. Fasting tends to normalize T4 production.

Testosterone levels can fall during fasting, although they will return to normal or prefast levels once fasting is completed. Serum melatonin and zinc levels both rise considerably. There is some evidence that this rise in serum melatonin helps alleviate insomniac conditions once the fast is broken.

Fasting and Healing

Fasting has been found to help a number of disease conditions, often permanently. In addition to the hypertension trial noted earlier, a number of intriguing clinical trials and studies have treated many disease conditions with fasting. Here are some of those findings.

- Fasting has been found effective in the treatment of Type II diabetes, often reversing the condition permanently.

- Because of its long-term effects on metabolism, fat stores in the body, leptin, and disease conditions associated with obesity, fasting has been found to be one of the most effective treatments for obesity.

- A number of studies have found that fasting is beneficial in epilepsy, reducing the length, number, and severity of seizures. Researchers at the Great Ormond Street Hospital in England have found that a high-fat or ketogenic diet significantly reduces the severity and occurrence of epileptic seizures in children. Such seizures have been linked to glucose metabolism, and speculation is that either too much sugar from a refined foods diet or improper glucose metabolism is at fault. By altering the body's glucose metabolism, shifting it to using ketone bodies as a fuel, seizures are either alleviated or eliminated in most children. Helen Cross, a pediatric neurologist who participated in the recent study, commented to BBC News that ketogenic diets "should be established as a recognized alternative treatment for any child with challenging or resistant epilepsy." Studies on fasting in the treatment of epilepsy, because the shift to ketone bodies is more pronounced during a fast, show even better outcomes that the high-fat or ketogenic diet.

- Fasting is exceptionally beneficial in chronic cardiovascular disease and congestive heart failure, reducing triglycerides, blood pressure, atheromas, and total cholesterol and increasing HDL levels.

- In a 1988 trial of 88 people with acute pancreatitis, fasting was found to work better than *any other* medical intervention. Neither nasogastric suction nor cimetidine were found to produce effects as beneficial as those from fasting. Symptoms were relieved irrespective of the etiology of the disease.

- A number of studies have found that fasting is effective for treating both osteoarthritis and rheumatoid arthritis. Fasting induces significant anti-inflammatory actions in the body, and researchers found decreased erythrocyte sedimentation rate (ESR), arthralgia, pain, stiffness, and need for medication.

- Autoimmune diseases such as lupus, rosacea, chronic urticaria, and acute glomerulonephritis have all responded well to fasting.

- Severe toxic contamination has been shown to be significantly helped by fasting. Clinical trials have found that people poisoned with PCBs (polychlorinated biphenyls) experienced "dramatic" relief after fasts of 7–10 days.

- Poor immune function improves during fasting. Studies have found that there is increased macrophage activity, increased cell-mediated immunity, decreased complement factors, decreased antigen-antibody complexes, increased immunoglobulin levels, increased neutrophil bactericidal activity, depressed lymphocyte blastogenesis, heightened monocyte killing and bactericidal function, and enhanced natural killer cell activity.

- Other diseases that have responded to fasting are psychosomatic disease, neurogenic bladder, psoriasis, eczema, thrombophlebitis, varicose ulcers, fibromyalgia, neurocirculatory disease, irritable bowel syndrome, inflammatory bowel disease, bronchial asthma, lumbago, depression, neurosis, schizophrenia, duodenal ulcers, uterine fibroids, intestinal parasites, gout, allergies, hay fever, hives, multiple sclerosis, and insomnia.

- The historical claim that fasting increases life span is beginning to garner some support in research literature. Regularly repeated 4-day fasting has been found to increase the life span in both normal and immunocompromised mice.

- Although the use of fasting in the treatment of cancer is controversial, there is some emerging data that fasting helps prevent cancer. Intermittent fasting (2 days weekly) has been shown to have an inhibitory effect on the development of liver cancer in rats.

Side Effects from Fasting

People experience a wide range of side effects during fasting, as follows. These seem to depend on the individual and his or her particular health picture. No one experiences all of these side effects during a fast.

- Dizziness, especially on standing quickly. This comes from the lower blood pressure that occurs during fasts. *It is important during water fasts to sit first if you have been lying down, then stand slowly near something you can hold on to.*
- Confusion and mental fog. This comes from the brain shift from glucose to ketones as fuel. It usually passes within 2–4 days.
- Cold extremities, sometimes unpleasantly so. This, like dizziness, is from the decreased blood pressure. Blankets are usually a necessity during deep fasting. Fasting in the winter is often more difficult because of the increased body coldness.
- Weakness. This is common on water fasts and will last throughout the fast. *Exercise other than occasional walking should be avoided on water fasts.* While gentle walking or bodily movement can often help an overall sense of well-being on a water fast, rigorous exercise of any sort makes energy demands on the body that can only be met by its use of protein for fuel. This will lead to much more muscle loss and can place a significantly heavier burden on your body. Rigorous exercise dur-

ing a water fast is strongly discouraged. Gandhi commented in his writings that his misunderstanding of this—he walked many miles each day on his first long water fast—caused him to seriously injure his body. He never completely recovered. This is a time to allow the body to conserve energy and go about the process of healing and detoxifying itself.

- Nausea. This is quite common and is often a component of the body processing the toxins that are stored in fat tissue. Nausea can often be alleviated by drinking more water.

- Occasionally some people experience vomiting. This can often be avoided by drinking lots of water (three to six 8 ounce cups daily). Vomiting, however, is sometimes a part of the body's detoxification. Although I hate it myself, vomiting often leads to a sense of freshness and revitalization once it has passed. Excessive vomiting should be dealt with cautiously. It may indicate a serious problem and can also lead to dehydration. Make sure you replace the fluids you lose if you do vomit by drinking more water.

- Headaches. These can sometimes be severe, *especially if you are a caffeine user*. Caffeine use should be tapered off over a period of several weeks prior to a fast to avoid this. Caffeine withdrawal can produce one of the truly great 1- or 2-day headaches of all time, especially if you drink lots of coffee. Most headaches pass in a day or two and are often helped by drinking more water.

- Coated tongue and bad breath. This is common. Normally the tongue will clear to a healthy pink color in

7–30 days, depending on how much work your body has to do to detoxify itself. *It is not necessary for the tongue to completely clear to have a successful fast.*

- Strong urine color and odor. The body is working to clear toxins and engage in deep healing. During this period the primary route of elimination are the kidneys. The urine will begin to clear as the fast progresses.
- Strong body odor. This may occur from the elimination of toxins from the skin during the fast.
- Metallic or other odd taste in the mouth. This comes from the ketones, especially acetone excreted through respiration, and will pass at the end of the fast. Usually after a few days you will become used to it.
- Lowered and/or feeble pulse. This is also from lowered blood pressure and altered cardiac activity.
- Severe gout. This can occur if your fluid intake falls below 1 cup of water per day.
- Emotional distress. This is often a component of fasting as the emotional and spiritual toxins emerge. It is important to work with them consciously.
- Little desire for sleep. As the fast progresses many people feel little desire for sleep at night. They may often want to catnap during the day instead. In many respects the lack of nighttime sleep is because your body is already in a sleep/resting mode. The sleep you do have at night during a fast then tends to focus on dreaming, an entirely different need from what fasting can provide. Once the dreaming is done, you have no more need for sleep. Sleep patterns normalize when the fast is broken. If you suffered from insomnia

prior to the fast, it will usually not recur after fasting,
unless you reimmerse yourself in the same conditions
that led to its original appearance.

- The reappearance of old disease symptoms. Normally
  this is the body attending to conditions that were not
  completely healed when they originally appeared.
  These usually appear in reverse order of their original
  occurrence.

- Joint, bone, or other localized pain in the body. The
  body acts to repair itself during fasts, and you may
  experience localized pain as it works on a particular
  area. I have noticed an increase in bone and joint pain
  as the people who attend my wife's and my vision
  quests age. Those over 45 seem most susceptible.
  While there is little or nothing in the literature on this,
  our working hypothesis is that it is the body repairing
  itself. The pain seems most localized to those places
  that are commonly the sites of arthritis or bone loss in
  aging populations: spine, hips, neck, and so on. While
  this pain can be severe, it generally begins to pass by
  the tenth to fourteenth day of longer fasts.

- Extreme hunger. This usually passes by the second,
  third, or fourth day of fasting. *It is very rare to be hungry on a water fast once your body has shifted to ketosis.*

- Diarrhea sometimes occurs during detoxification,
  especially between the second and third day. It is usually of short duration. Because you will be losing water
  if you have diarrhea, make sure you replace what is
  lost by drinking lots of water—at least 4–6 glasses
  (8 ounces each) per day.

- No bowel movements. Because there is no food intake, the need for bowel movements ceases. This is natural.

A Note on Enemas, Colonics, and Bowel Movements During Fasting

Normally, there are one or two bowel movements in the first three days of the fast as the colon eliminates the remains of prefast food intake. Thereafter bowel movements naturally cease. Occasionally, some people will have another one between 14 and 30 days into very long fasts. Rarely, some people will experience diarrhea in the initial days of the fast as their body is detoxing. It is important to monitor water intake if that occurs in order to make sure that dehydration is minimized. For those without diarrhea, a mild herbal laxative like senna tea *may* sometimes help fasting nausea early in the fast. Normally the bowel movement occurs 3–4 hours after the tea is consumed.

However, while enemas and colonics are often suggested by some proponents, and while the decision to utilize them is a personal one, there is little evidence to show that they actually do what they are purported to do.

A number of books on fasting show rather graphic photographs of the contents of bowels that have been flushed with enemas during fasting. Normally, it is asserted that these things are up inside people, should not be there, and are contributing to illness. So in a desire to get all the bad stuff out, enemas or colonics are suggested. Usually proponents find that these enemas need to be repeated regularly because more bad stuff is found as the fast progresses. An interesting discovery about this was made by a fasting researcher in 1907. He cleaned and then sequestered a portion of a faster's bowel. He found that the fecal-like material reappeared in a few days. The material that is being ejected with fasting enemas is in fact produced by the coevolutionary bacteria that line the large intestine. Most of the content of feces is really just this material. They produce it daily during their life cycle. Embedded within it, when the normal diet is ingested, are the unusable elements of the foods we eat such as fiber. The contents being ejected through enemas are in fact supposed to be there and are naturally produced by our bacterial partners, and we are evolutionarily designed to have it there. We are, after all, symbiotic beings on a symbiotic planet. Nevertheless, in some instances enemas may help—it is, in the end, a personal decision.

People Who Should Not Fast

Although most people can fast, there are a few who, because of special conditions, should not.

- People who are extremely emaciated or in a state of starvation
- Those who are anorexic or bulimic
- Pregnant, diabetic women
- Nursing mothers
- Those who have severe anemia
- Those with an extreme fear of fasting
- Those with porphyria. Porphyria refers to a genetic metabolic defect that affects the body's ability to manage porphyrins, a group of compounds that combine with iron to produce blood, are involved in the control

of electron transport systems, and, within mitochondria, are intricately involved in the production, accumulation, and utilization of energy. Porphyria can cause malfunctions in the liver, bone marrow, and red blood cells and produces a wide range of symptoms, including seizures.

- People with a rare, genetic, fatty acid deficiency that prevents proper ketosis from occurring. This is a deficiency involving the enzyme acetyl CoA, a mitochondrial fatty acid oxidation enzyme, that is essential to ketosis. Those with this deficiency who do fast can experience severe side effects, including hepatic steatosis, myocardial lipid accumulation, and severe hypoglycemia.

A Note on Pregnancy, Children, and Fasting

Although many fasting texts suggest that pregnant women not fast, those that have been found to suffer side effects have also been diabetic. Ketosis during pregnancy can seriously harm the fetus *if* the mother is diabetic. Fasting during pregnancy if a woman is not diabetic has not been found harmful to either mother or fetus. However, fasts for nondiabetic pregnant women should be no longer than 2–3 weeks' duration and should be monitored by a health care provider. Children, even infants, can also fast without complications if the fasts are relatively short—for infants, 2–3 days, and for children, 1–2 weeks, depending on age. These fasts should also be monitored by a health care provider unless they are short. The need for infants and young children to fast is rare. The most common condition indicating fasting for children is epilepsy.

Those Who Should Fast Under Health Care Supervision

While most people can fast safely, there are some who should do so only under the supervision of a health professional experienced in fasting for healing.

- Those with serious disease conditions
- Pregnant women
- Infants and young children
- Type I diabetics
- Those with insufficient kidney function
- Those who are extremely afraid of fasting yet wish to do so anyway
- People with a high toxic contamination level of DDT. This pesticide is stored by the body in a highly concentrated form in fat tissue. Fasting can release huge levels of DDT into the bloodstream as the fat stores are released. This can be quite dangerous.

Death During Fasting

Because so much fear about personal mortality and whether or not it is possible to live without eating can arise during fasting, here are some statistics about death and fasting.

Fasting is exceptionally safe, and death during fasting is extremely rare. I am aware of only 9 cases in the literature, a literature that covers hundreds of thousands of fasts over the past 125 years. Two of these occurred when the fasters ate heavy meals after very long fasts of 21 days or more—one man was fasting under an inexperienced physician's supervision and was following the protocol his physician had given him. Seven were suffering severe chronic disease conditions from which death was inevitable. They were fasting as a last attempt to heal themselves. In none of the cases was death attributable to the fast itself.

Juice Fasting

Although true fasting is a dry fast, without the consumption of anything at all, there are a number of specific kinds of non-dry fasts: porridge fasts, grape fasts, bread fasts, even the urine—more commonly known as the water of life—fast. The two primary forms of fasting practiced now, however, are water and juice fasting. Juice fasting is significantly different from water fasting. It has many benefits, and I personally like both water and juice fasts at different times for different reasons. Deep fasts are always water or dry fasts. They are indicated for those times when you want or need to work with the fundamental spiritual, emotional, and physical healing and detoxification that are necessary at times of great crisis, disease, or transition. Juice fasts are, as I noted earlier, a freshening or tuneup, or something to do when the demands of life do not allow a full immersion in deep, transformational fasting. Juice fasting is also extremely good for people who have never fasted before and want to test the waters and see just what they are getting themselves into. Juice fasts will help the body detoxify and heal to some extent, especially if they follow deep fasting and are repeated on a regular schedule. They will also provide a freshening of personal energy, an increase in physical and spiritual energy, and a better and more healthy relationship with food. They will also allow you to continue to work, to exercise, and to maintain daily energy levels.

More on the Physiology of Juice Fasting

Juice fasting is more properly a severely restricted diet. Because the fruits and vegetables are juiced and strained, the body has to do very little digestive work to assimilate the contents of the juice. These are broken apart in the various parts of the intestine and then transported quickly through the intestinal walls into the blood and then throughout the body. Normally, because there is significant carbohydrate content in these juices, the body does not go into a full state of ketosis. Ketosis is only partial as the body extracts fatty acids from fat stores to make up the difference between what it needs and what it is getting in the diet. Because ketosis is not complete, the physiological shifts that occur in ketosis either do not occur at all or do not occur completely. The body, for example, never drops completely into a state of rest, repair, and restoration. Benefits are correspondingly different. There is a cleaning and detoxification process that does occur because the load on the body has dropped considerably, allowing it to focus more attention on its healing. However, it never approaches the level of regeneration that can occur with deep fasting and is rarely as beneficial in the treatment of severe chronic disease conditions. Normally, hunger pangs do not disappear on a juice fast because the normal appetite suppressants that come into play once the body enters ketosis are not activated. One of these is orexin.

During the initial phases of fasting, the levels of orexin (also called hypocretin, or OX1R) in the hypothalamus and amygdala increase significantly. Orexin is actually a pair of hormones, released into the blood, that stimulate the desire to eat when blood sugar drops. This elevation of orexin stops after ketosis is fully initiated. During juice fasts the body is simply experiencing food deprivation, not complete fasting. It goes partly into ketosis but not fully, and so the body keeps producing orexin and other appetite stimulation hormones in order to motivate you to eat. This can make juice fasting much more difficult than water fasting—at least as far as hunger is concerned—because after the initial transition to ketosis occurs with water fasts, there is simply no desire for food.

However, one great benefit of juice fasting—or even modified juice fasting that utilizes special teas (I talk about these later in the book)—is that the juices can be intentionally chosen for their medicinal effects. This can produce significant healing in and of itself, if the right juices are chosen for the right conditions. (A list of the medicinal actions of various juices is included in appendix 2.)

Juice fasting is also: (1) exceptionally good as a way to first experience fasting; (2) crucial in moving from a modified diet into a full-blown water fast; and (3) extremely helpful while breaking a fast. It is often the case that the normal diet for most of us has not been all that healthy. During periods when someone wishes to do a deep fast, it is very important to begin with a lengthy low-fat organic diet to allow the body, mind, and spirit to begin to adjust to what is about to happen. Then the next stage is a juice fast, then a water fast; a juice fast should follow it, then a low-fat diet again.

Going from a very poor diet right into a water fast is very hard physically, emotionally, and spiritually. The amount of toxin release is increased substantially and concentrated within a short period of time. Modified diet and juice fasting allow the detoxification processes to occur incrementally, and the resulting toxin release during water fasting becomes much milder in its impacts.

Both types of fasting are great; they just do different things. Each is of benefit at different times, depending on what *you* want from your fast.

Physical Fasting and Friendship with the Body

In spite of all this detail about what fasting does in the body and how it does it, the fact that fasting is restorative, rejuvenative, and healing to many disease conditions, with strong impacts on levels of vitality and length of life, has been known for millennia. Fasters who hate the body, however, rarely can maintain such benefits. For the body is our first and best friend. It can be trained, as children and pets can be trained, but if its will is broken, just as when the spirits of children and pets are broken, the long-term outcome is always poor. Each of us is normally supposed to experience a wonderful and powerful joy that comes from deep in our bodies and flows outward. This can never occur if we treat our bodies with contempt. Clarissa Pinkola Estes comments:

> We tend to think of the body as this "other" that does its thing without us. Many people treat their bodies as if the body were a slave. We have only to pay heed to our bodies to know what we must do. The body is not sculpture

or marble. Its purpose is to protect, contain, support, and fire the spirit and soul within it, to be a repository for memory, to fill us with feeling.... The body is best understood as a being in its own right, one who loves us, depends on us, one to who we sometimes mother, and who sometimes is mother to us.[4]

When we consciously alter our and our body's relationship with food, we begin the often difficult process of making friends with our body and ourselves. We begin to trust what the body can do, and so we step back and let the body do what it has always been capable of doing. We allow it to go where it uniquely knows to go. We throw the reins on its neck and allow it to take us home. This can only happen if we come to love it, to be its friend, to honor what and who it is. It will never occur if we hate it, if we feel it is unclean or evil or an abode of sin. It is the first and best friend that the Universe has given to us, and it is through the body, not in spite of the body, that we find the luminous and the ineffable that our souls need to be whole.

5

Preparing for the Fast, Fasting, Breaking the Fast

The body is injured every time that one overeats, [or wrongly eats], and the injury can be partially repaired only by fasting.

— GANDHI

Two joys are prepared for him who observes the fast; the joy of breaking the fast and that of meeting his Lord.

— MOHAMMED

You will obtain better outcomes from your fast if the process is instituted slowly, with much thought and preparation beforehand. There are sixteen essential steps to every fast, as follows.

1. Determine if you are ready for a fast.
2. Decide what kind of fast is most supportive for you to do.
3. Arrange or set aside a special time for your fast.
4. Decide how long you are going to fast.
5. Arrange a supportive environment for the fast.
6. Begin eating a new diet to prepare your body for the fast for two to ten weeks prior to the fast.
7. If you are conducting your own fast, obtain good water and/or good foods to juice and drink during your fast.
8. Set your spiritual goals for the fast.
9. Set your emotional goals for the fast.
10. Set your physical goals for the fast.
11. Arrange sufficient time after the fast for you and your body to reintegrate and be ready for resuming daily life.
12. Keep a journal of your fast.
13. Fast with conscious attention to the process.
14. Break the fast with caring and awareness; especially make sure that you have the right kinds of foods on hand for breaking the fast.
15. After the fast, spend some time with someone who cares about you and whom you care about and tell this person about your experiences.
16. Incorporate the lessons of the fast into daily life.

Determine if You Are Ready for a Fast

Initially, the most important thing to consider is why you want to fast. You should fast because *you* want to, not because a voice in your head (or even in the room with you) is telling you that you will be better for it, more whole, cleaner, purer, or more spiritual. Fasting should be done because some deep part of your self lets you know that it is something you need to do to be who you are, who you want to be. The decision to fast often begins in a deep, unconscious part of the soul. It slowly gathers energy and, like a whale coming up for air, rises up one day all by itself into the conscious mind and lets you catch a glimpse of something of tremendous power and size. Then it submerges again. This starts the process of getting ready for the deep fast, it notifies the mind, emotions, the body, the entire self, that something difficult but life-altering is on the horizon. Like me, most people will not stop and heed its first message. That's the way it is with the conscious and unconscious. It lets us know something that we should do, and we ignore it until it won't let us do so anymore. So eventually it emerges again, farther out of the water, for longer, and perhaps its tail makes a huge splash just before it submerges again. Eventually, if we are smart, we begin to listen, to think, and to begin to prepare ourselves for a journey. Like all journeys, fasting takes preparation—preparation of the soul, the emotions, the body. The more conscious you are about what you are doing, the better prepared you will be and the more you will get from it.

Choose Your Fast

When you decide you are ready to fast, think about what kind of fast you want to do. Know also that the older you are, the more intense a fast can be, especially if you have been living a toxic lifestyle for a very long time. If you have never fasted before or if it has been a very long time since you have fasted, you should consider a juice fast—some of the juice blends that I think are very effective are listed in appendix 2. While a juice fast will, like a water fast, bring many benefits and will evoke many deep emotional, spiritual, and physical insights, it is much easier. A juice fast is the best way to first experience fasting. If you have fasted before or if you are working with an experienced fasting coach or health practitioner, then perhaps you will want to do a deep water fast. A water fast will be much more demanding; the degree of emotional, physical, and spiritual intensity is much higher. The benefits are correspondingly greater, but only if you are ready for it, and are not forcing yourself into it too quickly. While a water fast is exceptionally safe, *if you engage in a water fast before you are ready to do so, you risk doing yourself spiritual, emotional, and physical violence.* Neither fast is better or worse than the other, they just do different things. Each type of fast will make different demands on you; both are of great benefit.

Arrange or Set Aside Special Time for Your Fast

When you decide to fast, you begin to alter your basic relationship with food, emotional nurturing, survival, your body, your friends, your family, yourself, your culture, and your health. It can stir up many things. Fasts are most effective if you give some thought to when the most supportive time for your fast might be. What is the best time of year? When will the demands on your life be less stressful? Do you need to go on a special retreat in the wilderness for your fast? Or do you feel it would be better if you went to a special retreat center that specializes in fasting? If you are going to go away for your fast, when can you really take the time to do so? All these things should be taken into account. You should give it all the thought it deserves and pick a time that you feel will be the most supportive of what you want to accomplish. Once you have decided that you are going to fast, the type of fast, and when you are going to fast, the process of the fast begins. All of your being will be readying itself for the fasting time to come.

Decide How Long You Are Going to Fast

It is crucial to decide for how long you are going to fast before you begin. The part of you that wants to eat will feel more taken care of if it knows just how long you will be fasting. It is important as well that you keep your word to yourself and only fast just this long. Once you are an experienced faster, that part of you will trust you more, knowing that food will come again, that you will not starve, and that many wonderful benefits will come from fasting; at that time it is possible to decide on a more open-ended fast. If you are new to fasting, start with a short fast and let yourself get used to the process. Use the following guidelines to help you determine the length of time you should fast. (Water fasts for serious disease conditions often need to be longer; the length of time

Fasting Time Guidelines

WATER FASTING

Regular diet
2 weeks (minimum) low-fat cleansing diet
3 days fresh juices and herbal teas only
4–10 days water only
1–3 days fresh juices; miso soup; mild,
    heavily steamed vegetables
4–14 days low-fat cleansing diet
Regular diet

(The length of time spent on each of these sections depends on a person's physical, emotional, and spiritual condition and needs. NOTE: For every day of a water fast, there should be one day of recovery. If you spend 10 days on a water fast, you should spend at least 10 days recovering before engaging in intensive activity.)

JUICE FASTING

Regular diet
2 weeks (minimum) low-fat cleansing diet
4–30 days fresh juices and herbal teas only
1 day miso soup and mild, heavily
    steamed vegetables
4–14 days low-fat cleansing diet
Regular diet

(The length of time spent on each of these sections depends on a person's physical, emotional, and spiritual condition and needs.)

should be determined in consultation with a health care provider experienced in fasting for healing.)

Arrange a Supportive Environment for the Fast

Choose where you want to have your fast. The kind of fast you are doing will determine, to some extent, where you can do it. If you are going into the wilderness for a deep water fast retreat, it is often good to go with a guide or a group of people engaged in similar deep wilderness fasting. You should find a guide or group you feel good about. If you are going to a special retreat center that offers fasting retreats, do some research and find one that you feel will be the most nurturing and caring. (There are some suggestions in the resources section.)

If you are juice fasting, which again, for me, includes lemonade/ maple syrup fasts, your daily environment will often still work, but it can need some slight alterations to make the fast as beneficial and supportive as possible.

You will need a good juicer if you are actually going to juice vegetables and fruits. You will need to obtain enough of the vegetables and juices for the length of time you are fasting. This is a retreat time, and it is most supportive if you can avoid supermarkets and other high-intensity/fluorescent-light environments as much as possible. Everything you need should already be available before the fast so that all you have to do is concentrate on the fast itself. If you are using a lemonade/maple syrup fast, then all of those ingredients should be on hand, enough for the entire fast. Make sure you buy only organic ingredients. You are fasting for detoxification and physical cleansing, and it will be easier on your body if you give it the cleanest, healthiest juice you can. Buy your own vegetables and fruits. When you pick them out, attend to them. Choose the ones you feel, for whatever reason, are the happiest, brightest, healthiest—the ones that seem to glow most. Even if the difference is a tiny one, pay attention to it.

Next choose how you want each day to be during the fast. If you are doing a juice fast and are intending to work, be prepared for what you will tell your coworkers about your changed diet. It is best if you can tell them nothing at all. It cannot be stressed enough that the food issues that the people around you have will be activated by your fasting. It is extremely common for people on a fast to receive a great deal of unwanted advice, warnings, and jokes about fasting from those around them. The simplest thing to do is to go off by yourself for awhile during lunch and drink juice you have prepared for yourself before you left home. You will get much more out of the fast if you prepare all of your juice yourself instead of buying it readymade, even if it is from a fresh juice bar. There is an essential relationship with food that a fast reveals. Choosing the foods and preparing them yourself are important and highly meaningful elements of the juice fast. You are giving a gift to yourself, one that you will receive more easily if it comes from your own hands.

If you can't avoid telling your coworkers what you are doing, tell them your doctor wanted you to go on this diet for 10 days or for whatever length of time you have decided to fast. Give them a wry grin and shrug as if you have little say in the matter. If they think you *have* to do it, they will be much less likely to offer unwanted advice or suggestions. If you are lucky, your coworkers will know about fasting, and you can share freely about what you are doing.

If you have a family you live with, you may want to sit down with them and tell them you are going to be fasting and ask for their support. You should know up front that it is much more difficult to fast when the people around you are eating. The smell of the food and your family's obvious enjoyment and intimate sharing during the preparation and eating of the food will make it more difficult—you may feel left out. You will have to be very clear about what you are doing, why you are doing it, and for how long. You should clearly realize that when you fast, you are breaking a number of often unconscious agreements you have with your family about food and nurturing. You should clearly consider if they will be able to be supportive. If not, it is much kinder on yourself and them to fast someplace else. Sometimes, the appearance of fasting within the family as it goes about its daily tasks is just too confrontive to the underlying family agreements, assumptions, and emotional stroke patterns that all of you have around food.

Make sure during the fast that your physical surroundings are as relaxing as possible. Make sure, as much as you can, that you will not have to deal with any highly stressful demands during your fast. Create a structure that allows you to feel as nurtured as possible. During your fast, arrange things so that you can avoid doing housework, paying bills, working around the house, talking to contractors, or going to court. Make this a special time for you as much as you can. The more supportive, nonstressful time you can give yourself, the more you will receive from the fast.

If you are water fasting, the environment is much more important, as the demands of the fast are much higher. You will not be able to work on a water fast; *you must take time off from work*. While water fasts can occur in your normal residential setting, your sensitivity to formerly unnoticed events will increase substantially. Normal background noise of living in a city or town can be highly stressful on a water fast. Family members walking through the room 10 times in an hour can be irritating. Television is simply dreadful, cooking smells nauseating, perfume and fingernail polish like being locked inside a chemical factory, and the steady, hour-long stare of your dog as you lie weakly helpless on the couch truly infuriating. It can be done, but you will find it much less stressful and significantly more supportive if you find a place for retreat. A wilderness setting or fasting retreat center is often best.

I have spent such retreat time in the high Rocky Mountains, in Christian monasteries, in a kiva in the ground, and at retreat centers. All of them have their benefits and drawbacks. My overall preference is for wilderness settings, though a close second is an isolated retreat center that has been crafted with caring and loving attention. Whatever place you choose, make sure that to the deep part of you that wants to fast it feels good. Make sure that some part of you says "Yes, this will work." Make sure that at the place you choose, if there are other people involved, they know what you are doing and are supportive of it. There are a great many spiritual retreat centers throughout the world that support transformational water and juice fasting. There are also many centers that specialize in supervising water fasts (see the references section for some ideas). Know that if you water fast at home, all the things said here about juice fasting will apply, trebled at least.

Whatever kind of fast you do, your environment should feel as supportive and loving as possible.

Begin Eating a New Diet to Prepare Your Body for the Fast

Some of the factors that can increase the intensity of your fast are:

1. If you have never fasted before
2. If it has been a very long time since you fasted
3. If you are middle-aged or older
4. If you are in a difficult life transition
5. If you are doing a deep, spiritual, wilderness fast
6. If you eat a diet high in refined foods
7. If you have been under high stress for some time
8. If you have high levels of toxins in your body (if your job entails any contact with synthetic chemicals on a regular basis, you will have a high toxin load)
9. If you have taken a lot of pharmaceuticals during your life

The more of these things that are true, or the more intensely they are true, the longer you should eat a preparation diet before fasting and the more carefully you should prepare emotionally and spiritually for the fast. This especially includes carefully considering your emotional relationship with food. To help prepare both your body and mind, I suggest that you eat a low-fat cleansing diet (see appendix 1) for a minimum of 2 weeks prior to fasting; the longer you follow this diet, the easier the fast will be. If you eat similarly to this diet most of the time, then one to two weeks is enough. Then go into a juice fast, then water fast (if you are water fasting), then back to the juices, then back to the cleansing diet, then to the regular diet if desired. If you are going to do a water fast, do the juice fast for 3 days after the cleansing diet before going to the water fast.

If you are currently taking pharmaceuticals, if at all possible, they should be discontinued during the fast. If possible they should be discontinued during the prefast diet. If you are taking pharmaceuticals for a serious illness and you cannot eliminate them, you should consider doing a healing fast under medical supervision. During the fast you should plan on taking no vitamin or herbal supplements (except for juices if you are juice fasting) and no over-the-counter medications such as aspirin. Fasts allow your body to engage in the healing processes it needs; foreign substances make that process more difficult.

If You Are Conducting Your Own Fast, Obtain Good Water and/or Good Foods to Juice and Drink During Your Fast

Make sure you use only healthy spring water for your fast. Do not use distilled water. Distilled water has been technologically altered, and many if not most of the minerals and nutrients have been removed. Do *not use tap water.* Use the healthiest, wildest, most natural water you can.

Again, if you are juicing on this fast, obtain only organic vegetables and fruits. Pick them out yourself from a market that feels good and nurturing to you, and choose the ones that seem most alive and healthy to you.

You are giving yourself a gift; make sure that the contents of the gift are ones that you feel good about receiving. If you have had a long and not terribly good relationship with food, use the foods you choose for the cleansing diet and the ones for juicing as an opportunity for beginning a new kind of relationship with food. Choose with awareness, choose with caring, choose with love.

Set Your Spiritual Goals for the Fast

The first and most important thing in preparing yourself for a fast is to think about what you want to receive from it, *why* you are doing it. The more clearly you can define your goals, the more conscious you will be during the fast and the more you will gain from it. Before you do so, however, ask yourself these important questions about your relationship with your spiritual life.

1. When you were growing up, what and who did you want to be?
2. How close to this goal are you now?
3. Have you ever felt that you were born for a particular reason, and if so, what is it?
4. How do you feel when you consider what you thought you were to become and when you consider what you have now become?
5. Is there any relationship between how you perceive your body, how you use food, and this feeling?
6. Have you ever had the sense that the world around you is magical, alive, luminous, and deeply sacred or mysterious?
7. How long has it been since you experienced this feeling?
8. How did your family talk about your purpose in the world, and about what you would probably become, when you were growing up?

9. What unspoken agreements existed between you and your family about your purpose in the world in this lifetime?

10. Was it okay within your family for you to have a spiritual self and a life's work?

11. How would they feel if you allowed your spiritual self to emerge?

12. How do you think that your coworkers would feel and act if you allowed your spiritual self to emerge?

13. How do you think that your culture and local community would act and feel if you allowed your spiritual self to emerge?

14. What would have to change in your life if you gained a sense of your spiritual purpose during fasting and decided to follow it?

15. Do you think you would be willing to do it?

16. What is missing from your life?

Think deeply about these things, for any truths that are underneath these questions are inside you and can emerge during fasting. Once you have thought deeply about these questions, then, and only then, decide and write down in as much detail as you can why you are going to be engaging in a deep fast. What spiritual outcomes do you want, what spiritual food are you seeking? If you could gain any spiritual outcome you wish from your fast, what would it be?

Set Your Emotional Goals for the Fast

You may find, upon thinking about why you are fasting, that your relationship with food is unhealthy. As an initial part of experiencing a healthy fast, you may decide that you need to overcome some of your unhealthy relationships with food. Although it seems antithetical to fasting, you may find that if, for a time, you allow yourself to eat whatever you want, your body will eventually start to want very different foods from those you have been eating: greens, fruits, and specific proteins. The body has its own wisdom, and once you can hear what it is saying, have shown that you are willing to listen to what it is telling you, it will begin notifying you when it needs fruits, salads, soups, meats, or sugars. Once you reestablish this trust between yourself and your body, what happens is that your desire for certain kinds of food will go way down, and for others, way up. The decision has to be a real one, though. You cannot fake it in the hopes that you will eventually *only* want "good" food. The first step is to eat *exactly* what you want. If it is ice cream for breakfast, omelets for dinner, steak and potatoes for lunch, do it. Your body will also tell you when it has had enough. All living beings have a natural response to having eaten sufficient food. A baby turns its head from its mother's breast when it is full. It is only after we have been taught an unhealthy relationship with food that we continue to eat after we are full. As Carol Normandi and Laurelee Roark comment in their book *It's Not About Food,*

> to try and weed out what society tells us about food and what our bodies tell us about food requires the radical approach of "legalizing" all foods. No food is bad, and no food is good. Candy, avocados, pasta and celery are all

equal. The only difference is how your own body feels after eating a particular food. . . . Our own bodies are the
best at telling us what we should and should not eat, not
the culture, not the "diet experts," not the television commercials and the magazine ads, and not our own minds
that have been brainwashed on what is "good."[1]

[For] when you stop defining a food as "bad" or
"wrong" or "unattainable" or "fattening," you can start
seeing it objectively as just another food with a certain
shape, taste, and physical effect on your body.[2]

If you "insist" that your body begin eating only "good" foods
or stop eating others that you define as "bad," you initiate an internal experience of deprivation; and the primary response to
deprivation of the body, of that part of you that is in charge of
your food survival, is binging.

If you feel, however, that you are ready for a fast—that your
relationship with food is healthy enough to actually fast—begin
looking at your emotional world and its relationship to food. Ask
yourself these important questions:

1. Let yourself remember your earliest memories of
   food. What are they?
2. What feelings come up when you remember these
   early memories?
3. What other memories about food come up?
4. What feelings do you have about them?
5. What can't you stand allowing yourself to feel?
6. What unspoken agreements do you and your family
   have about food?

7. Are there any feelings that you use food to make go away?
8. What happened to you in your family when you were wrong?
9. How do you feel about your body the way it is now?
10. If you are thinner, do you believe you will be more loved?
11. If you lose weight, do you believe you will be happier?
12. In general, how do you feel about food?
13. Were you breast fed?
14. What stories were you told by your family about your first year of life and your relationship with food? with bottles? with breastfeeding?
15. What feelings come up when you think about yourself, as an infant, breastfeeding?

Again, think deeply about these things, for any truths that are underneath these questions are inside you and can emerge during fasting. Once you have thought deeply about these questions, then, and only then, decide what your emotional goals are from fasting. If you could have any emotional outcome you want from fasting, what

> A genuine fast cleanses body, mind, and soul.
> —GANDHI

would it be? As you think on these things, consider as well: What concerns and fears arise when you think about fasting? What, in fact, is your greatest fear about fasting? If you have concerns that are not addressed by this book, spend some time researching fasting and see if you can find an answer to those concerns. It is important that the part of you that is concerned with your survival feels that you have done everything necessary to ensure your safety during the fast.

Set Your Physical Goals for the Fast

Consider the following questions before you set your physical goals.

1. Do you believe that your body can be healthy?
2. Do you think that the body is made to fast?
3. Do you believe that your body has an innate wisdom that can actually guide it where it needs to go?
4. How healthy, actually, do you think your body is?
5. Can you conceive of your body as your friend?
6. What would it take for you and your body to be friends?
7. Do you have any beliefs about your body that may stand in the way of allowing it to become healthy?
8. Are there any illnesses that have been troubling you that you would like to see resolved?
9. Do you think it is possible to be healthy long into old age?
10. Do you like the way your body looks?
11. If not, do you blame your body for how it looks?
12. Can you conceive of your body as sacred?
13. How does it feel to believe that your body is sacred?

14. Let yourself sit and get comfortable. Then imagine, standing in front of you, the ugliest part of your body. How do you feel seeing this part of you? Look carefully at this part of you; what messages do you tell it every day? Is there something that this part of you wants to tell you? Is there something it wants from you? How do you feel about what it wants and says to you?

15. Are any of your physical or health problems located in this part of your body?

Once again, think deeply about these things, for any truths that are underneath these questions are inside you and can emerge during fasting. Once you have thought deeply about these questions, then, and only then, decide what your physical goals are for your fast.

As an aside: the physical goals you set should not be of the order of goals like "I will lift 200 pounds 20 times each day to help me get in shape." In other words, the goals should not be related to any kind of boot camp or "should" kinds of thinking. These goals are more supportive if they are of the order of things like: *I want my body to feel healthier than before the fast. I want to love my body more. I want to be healed in this area of my body.*

Most of us are trained out of perceiving our bodies as holy, trained instead to see our bodies in distorted and misguided ways, to distrust their impulses, even to believe they have our worst interests at heart rather than our best. We have learned to believe that the human body is just like the rest of physical creation—is merely matter, dumb, unintelligent, and uncaring. When you begin the difficult task of ceasing hostilities with your body, begin to listen to it and trust it, you directly confront the most basic beliefs you have been given about your physical self. It is one of the most loving and most powerful acts of courage and faith that you can do.

Arrange Sufficient Time After the Fast for Reintegration

It takes one additional recuperation day for every day of a water fast to recover from fasting. If you water fast for 7 days, you will need 7 days after the fast to recover. Juice fasting is easier. If you juice fast for 7 days, you will only need 1 or 2 days for recovery. If you are a first-time faster, you will need 2 or 3 days of recovery and reintegration time after a juice fast. Make sure you give yourself the gift of this time; allow this extra time when you are figuring out the time span needed for your fast. *This recuperation time is as important as the fast itself.* You will experience a number of important changes in your body, mind, and spirit during the fast. Often these changes are deeper and more substantial than you know and will only become clear when you are once again entering your daily life and once more interacting with the people, and foods, that are normally a part of your life. The contrast between how you are now, after the fast, and how the rest of your life still is will make plain just how much you have changed. So allow all of yourself, your body, mind, and spirit, to have time to adjust. It is an extreme act of kindness to give yourself this integration time. What you take away from your fast will be the better for it.

Keep a Journal of Your Fast

A journal is important during a fast. It gives you a direct outlet for the many experiences you are having. Scores of thoughts, feelings, discomforts, and insights will occur while you are fasting. If you give yourself a medium in which to express them, some of the internal pressure of these events can be lessened. With a journal, the intensity has an outlet.

A journal also gives you a written record of your movement through the fast; it is a description of the terrain of your journey. You are going into an uncharted land, a unique territory of the human spirit, the emotional self, and the body. The content of this written record will often amaze you when you later revisit it. Without a journal, many of the insights will be difficult to remember consciously when you return to your regular life. They can even be hard to remember at later stages of the fast.

Fast with Conscious Attention to the Process

When you are fasting, pay special attention to each moment. Long periods of water fasting are very boring. There is little to do and even less strength to do it. Most of the time is spent lying around *experiencing* the fast. In spite of this, work to stay with the process. Allow yourself to watch what is happening to you as if you were a disinterested observer. Watch not only when your thoughts turn to food but just *how* they turn to food. Notice what feelings you have when you cannot eat. Are there feelings coming up that you would normally stuff down with food? Notice just what happens to you and your body when you consciously decide not to eat. What does it take for you to learn to eat the landscape around you instead of food? How does it feel to eat the landscape? Are there recurring thoughts and memories emerging, now that you have stopped eating, that have a source in your childhood? If you feel depressed, sit with the depression and try to trace it back to its source. When was the first time you felt this way? How long has it been since you allowed yourself to look at this particular depression?

As the fast progresses, do things begin to appear in a new light? Is there a special luminosity to the environment around you? Is there intelligence and soul there? As Hazrat Inayan Khan says most beautifully, "everything in life is speaking in spite of its apparent silence." Notice what the life around you is saying. How long has it been since you listened to the world speak? Notice your dreams as well; write them down and think about them during the long days of fasting.

You are engaged in a journey of change. *Everything* that happens on this journey has meaning; *everything* is a communication to you about the things you are fasting for. If you do not listen, you let a great life opportunity pass by. The more you attend to the fast with conscious awareness, the more you will gain from it.

Break the Fast with Caring and Awareness

If you have fasted in a retreat setting, make sure that the place you return to is comfortable and supportive. You will not have the energy to deal with problems or drama of any kind. The place needs to be restful—you should have to do nothing but be there. If you have spent time in a powerful wilderness setting, make sure that you have nothing to do for at least 2 days afterward; this especially includes driving in traffic. Make sure that your reintegration is slow, thoughtful, and cognizant of your increased sensitivities. If your fast has been a long one, make sure that you have at least 4 days, preferably a week, to reintegrate. Remember, you will need one day for each day you fasted to recover.

If you have deep fasted at home, make sure that you will not be disturbed as you begin breaking the fast. If you have done a deep fast of 7 days or less, make sure that nothing needs your attention for at least 2 days—at least 4 days if the fast was longer.

Reintegrate into food by reversing the eating patterns you used in preparing for the fast. Concentrate on juices and miso soups for at least 3 days. Slowly work back into the 10-week low-fat diet. Do not eat meat for at least 1 week.

When you are finished with the period of time you set aside for fasting and are ready to take food into your body again, it is most important to do so with great awareness. Make sure the foods you begin eating—spiritual, emotional, physical—are nurturing foods, and take them in slowly so that you can get used to them once again.

Carefully choose the physical food with which you are going to break the fast. Allow yourself to savor its preparation. Let your awareness focus on everything about it when you begin to eat it: its smell, its texture, its taste, how it feels in your body, and how your body reacts to it. Notice how incredibly nourishing this food *feels* as you take it inside you. Immerse yourself in the experience and truly receive the gift of this nurturing substance that so many people have worked for, that the Earth has provided, that is filled with the life that you need to continue on.

Remember: your entire digestive system has stopped its normal functioning during the fast. It is in a state of hibernation; it is turned off. It needs mild foods at first so that it can slowly come back on-line again. As you take in miso soup or freshly squeezed orange juice, the body and the digestive system begin to wake up again. Digestive enzymes once again start to be produced, and the whole physiology of the body begins to shift from ketosis back to glucose metabolism. Your brain begins to use a different food once more. All your body systems begin to shift in their orientation and performance. Allow them, and you, to take all the time necessary to make this change. Break the fast with very good food. *Slowly*. The more you allow your body to set the pace, the more healthy it will be and the more healthy your daily relationship with food will be. At this time you will notice an extreme sensitivity to food. Your vomeronasal organ will be exquisitely sensitive to the chemicals it encounters. You will be extremely sensitive to its messages. Your cells and organs will want particular food, unique to you, and if you listen carefully you will be able to determine just what you do want and what you do not. You may have spent days thinking about steak and ice cream. It is very rare that on finishing a fast anyone really wants those things. It often turns out that those thoughts were only coming from a part of you that was expressing the face of unmet desire. Usually, they are not an expression of what your deep self really needed or wanted. Let the wisdom of your body begin to guide you; trust it. In any event, you should not eat heavy foods on finishing a fast. Your digestive system, your entire body, is not ready to process that kind of food. The body needs at least 3 days to shift over to regular food intake, and even then the amounts desired and needed are usually tiny in comparison to your former meal intake.

If your fast has been a lengthy one, you will still be weak for some time. Give yourself the gift of letting your strength return in its own time. As you reintegrate and ingest more good food, it will come more and more quickly each day.

It is important that the part of you that loves and needs food feels cared for and supported. After all, you have just asked it to give up one of the things that is central to its purpose. It will always support you if you make sure that you care for it and its needs as well. This kindness toward this part of you, toward yourself, prepares you for "the holy communion of breaking bread with your self."

Spend Some Time After the Fast with Someone Who Cares About You

Once you have finished fasting, it is important to have people who understand what you have been doing welcome you back. Don't talk too much immediately on your return; leave yourself a day to get used to being in the presence of people again, to feel what it is like to have the energy that comes from them flow to you and into you. Just allow yourself to sit and feel what it is like to be coming back into the world.

After you have rested, perhaps that night or the next morning, it is good to share your story with those you have come back to. It is good to have the tale of the journey received by someone who cares and who, perhaps, can see or sense the deeper spiritual and emotional journey you have just made. This is your special time of reintegration, and it is important that this person focus on you and truly receive your sharing.

You have been on a journey. You have seen unusual things, had unusual experiences, perhaps struggled with unique obstacles. One of the most important things on returning from a journey is to share that journey with someone important to you, someone who loves you and whom you love. You have challenged your basic relationships with food, survival, your childhood messages about self-worth and nurturing, and your own spiritual destiny, and perhaps you have altered the very fabric of your deepest being. There are, perhaps, many things that you experienced that you can only understand if someone who loves you reflects them back. So take some time and sit with a good friend and tell him or her of your journey. Have your journal with you so that you can refer back to your record of the journey. Having someone receive the story of your journey shows your deepest self that this new relationship to food extends not only to those that you prepare for your body but also those that come from the hearts and hands of friends.

You have also been on a spiritual exploration of the meaning of your life and the deepest aspects of your essential self and the work you are here to do. Having someone receive the sharing of your increased awareness of those things, someone who offers support for your deepened commitment or awareness of your essential life work, is an extremely innervating experience. You have worked with the deepest and most vulnerable parts of yourself during your fast. You have perhaps taken the first trembling steps into the work you have been born to do. The loving and caring support of a good friend is essential at this moment in your life. As Chief Dan George put it:

> My friends, how desperately we need to be loved and to love. When Christ said that man does not live by bread alone, he spoke of a hunger. This hunger was not the hunger of the body. It was not the hunger for bread. He spoke of a hunger that begins deep down in the very

depths of our being. He spoke of a need as vital as breath. He spoke of the hunger for love.

Love is something you and I must have. We must have it because our spirit feeds upon it. We must have it because without it we become weak and faint. Without love our self-esteem weakens. Without it our courage fails. Without love we can no longer look out confidently at the world. We turn inward and begin to feed upon our own personalities, and little by little we destroy ourselves.

With it we are creative. With it we march tirelessly. With it, and with it alone, we are able to sacrifice for others.[3]

Incorporating the Lessons of the Fast into Daily Life

You may find that during the fast you traveled into the apparent emptiness of the desert and found a food that is tremendously filling, only to return to a home of seeming abundance that is devoid of filling food. Your heart and soul are filled, but there are dysfunctions—emotional toxins—that you can now clearly see within your family. As you begin reintegrating yourself into your life, notice the patterns there that you are now sensitive to. Notice what kinds of emotional food, emotional messages, you are receiving. Do you like them or not? Is there other food you would prefer? This is the time to begin working to integrate the lessons of the deep fast into your emotional world. How do you want to feel each day? What will it take to feel that way? What will it take to begin altering your family and daily life in such a way that the emotional food you need is abundant and filling?

Notice also the spiritual setting in which you find yourself. Does the luminosity that you found during the fast begin to fade? Remember any new or invigorated sense of direction you gathered to yourself during the fast. How can you, every day, incorporate some of this into your life?

Those parts of you that deep fasted to seek a better food, those deep soul parts of you, will be happier—you will be happier—if you consciously work to integrate the learnings of your fast into your daily life on a regular basis.

A Note on Repeated Fasting

Many people, once they have experienced the benefits of fasting, decide to repeat the experience. Long historical human experience with fasting and recent research have shown that fasting each year or at most every other year conveys tremendous benefits to physical health, spiritual and emotional well-being, and longevity. However, there are some potential problems with repeated fasting; the root of them is usually the reason why fasting is regularly repeated.

Again, you should repeat a fast because *you* want to, not because some outside authority or an internalized voice is telling you that you will be better, more whole, more clean, purer, or more spiritual if you do. Fasting is something that you should do *only* because some deep part of you knows it is what you need and you actually want to do it. The part of you that tells you the things you should do to be good is *not* the part of you that should determine whether or how often you should fast. Fasting needs to be attended to with the whole attention of the soul and all the unconscious and conscious parts of the self. If it is done for the wrong reasons, for appearance's sake, you will often do harm to yourself and gain very little from the fast.

Both Al-Ghazzali and Gandhi had succinct comments on repeated fasting. Al-Ghazzali said that by engaging in continual fasting the faster "departs from the established practice of the Apostle and makes fasting a yoke for himself although God would like him to enjoy his liberties just as much as He would want him to fulfil his obligations."[4] And Gandhi, that most accomplished faster, said: "I have also found that frequent fasting tends to rob it of its efficacy, for then it becomes almost a mechanical process without any background of thought. Every fast therefore should be undertaken after due deliberation."[5]

Repeated fasting can become an abuse of the body for those who see the body as an enemy of the spirit. The Puritan tradition runs very deep in the West, especially in America. This tradition has a deep suspicion of the body; there is a feeling that the flesh is evil, the body a tempter of the soul, and that the Earth is a pollution of the sacred. This strain of thought affects most all of us one way or another. In fasting it most often comes out as a desire to "cleanse" the body of all contaminants so that it is finally pure. In consequence some people engage in repeated fasts in an attempt to subdue the body, to purge its contamination of the soul. This is really an aberration of fasting, a historically more recent perspective on the nature of incarnation in physical form, and is in opposition to the inherent sacredness of the body and the manifestation of spirit as matter. The underlying attitudes and beliefs that motivate the act of fasting, as with any act, determine the outcome of the act. The reduction to technique of any inherently spiritual act is potentially dangerous, as the most important thing is the intent behind the act, *not* the act itself. Hugging someone when the heart is cold and dead to them is not a hug but something else entirely. Fasting when it is motivated by hatred of the body, a belief that it is impure and an impediment to the spirit's communion with the sacred, is not fasting but a violence to the deepest self and a desecration of the only home in the Universe that has been prepared especially for you.

The body has an intelligence and sacredness of its own. If you treat it with hatred it will respond as do all lovers—with rage. Only if you come to know it, to care for it and its ways, can you know the difference between what it needs and what it simply desires. If you honor and love the body, it will repay you in kind.

6

Deepening the Fast

A journey makes us vulnerable, takes us from our more secure environments and commits us to the unknown. Perhaps this is why the journey has so often been our basic metaphor for life itself. Our life journey is a precarious pilgrimage, a passage through landscapes of promise and peril, a crossing from the darkness of the womb to the shadows of death. We travel in the hope that the light will not fail to guide us, that the star will not be lost, that homecoming will be granted and love not withheld.

— THOMAS MERTON

Our religious beliefs separate heaven and earth, this life and the afterlife, and our philosophical thinking cuts apart mind and matter, all of which forces a chasm between the visible and the invisible . . . mysticism unites visible and invisible; all things are transparent and proclaim their invisible ground.

— JAMES HILLMAN

Fasting can become an intentionally spiritual act—an act that opens us to the touch of the sacred, opens deeper realms of the self to our inspection, allows us to sharpen normally atrophied capacities of perception, and allows the knowledge of our unique purpose to once again flow into our consciousness.

Without a sense of personal calling, life often seems, and is, empty. When you possess, at the very deepest levels of your being, the experience, the understanding, that there is a reason why you are alive and that you are wanted for the unique gifts only you can bring, life begins to take on a value of supreme depth and richness. There is a profound joy in such knowledge and a corresponding recognition that however dark some experiences may be, there is no place so dark that someone or something has not already been there before you and prepared your place—for each of these experiences contains some lesson for the development of the soul. Without them it is impossible to become who we are meant to be. All of us have intimations of this as we travel through our lives. All of us sense that, as Henry David Thoreau described it, we are applewood tables filled with eggs:

> Everyone has heard the story that has gone the rounds of New England, of a strong and beautiful bug which came out of the day leaf of an old table of apple-tree wood, which had stood in a farmer's kitchen for sixty years, first in Connecticut, and afterwards in Massachusetts,—from an egg deposited in the living tree many years earlier still, as appeared by counting the annual layers beyond it; which was heard gnawing out for several weeks, hatched perchance by the heat of an urn. Who does not feel his faith in resurrection and immortality strengthened by

hearing of this? Who knows what beautiful and winged life, whose egg has been buried for ages under many concentric layers of woodenness in the dead dry leaf of society, deposited at first in the alburnum of the green and living tree, which has been gradually converted into the semblance of its well-seasoned tomb,—heard perchance gnawing out now for years by the astonished family of man, as they sat round the festive board,—may unexpectedly come forth from amidst society's most trivial and handselled furniture, to enjoy perfect summer life at last![1]

All of us, under the years-long pressures of society, family, career, and youthful misunderstanding, tend to surround the winged part of ourselves in this kind of woodenness. We become stable, of a certain size and shape, reliable, predictable, fixed. Our winged life is dormant, encased in the woodenness of our lives. Sometimes there is a part of us that feels this, that describes our life as feeling "stuck."

We are called into this world; our being is not an accident. Our winged self is meant to take flight, to gnaw itself free from the woodenness of life. There is a deep, and powerful, part of us that knows this, knows that life is filled with meaning, knows that there are powers greater than ourselves that are here to help us on our way in the fulfillment of our unique destinies. Throughout each of our lives, this deep part of us, and the other powers that care deeply for our welfare, offers us glimpses of that destiny, offers us the knowledge that there is a winged self that only needs the heat of a fire to awaken it. As the woodenness of life grows thicker, we often encounter awakening fires with greater frequency, each possessing greater heat. For it is our destiny to awaken. We are always surrounded by messages to help us in this awakening. They reside deep within the world around us: odd experiences, brief glimpses of the luminous nature of things, unique feelings, the unusual glance in an old one's eyes, strange coincidences, unexplainable turnings of the wheel of life.

As we encounter the touches of our deep self, of the powers meant to help us on our way, we are being asked to become aware of something essential. The great analyst Victor Frankl said that there comes a time in each person's life when they walk out under the stars, look up at the sky, and ask, "God, what is the purpose of my life?" They almost always do so without realizing that they are not the questioner but the questioned. This question that we are being asked—unless we have already answered it—remains a constant all during life; the urging for its answer intensifies during the great transitions of our lives: adolescence, middle age, old age, and death. At each moment of our lives we have the opportunity to stop and grapple with it, to come to terms, to see the winged self within us and to begin setting it free. We can intentionally encounter this question, intentionally seek a great transition, intentionally place ourselves where we can meet the deeper parts of ourselves, the powers that are concerned with our welfare. We can go into the wilderness and fast. During such deep fasts we place ourselves next to a fire of great intensity. The heat of this urn can often awaken to life the egg long buried inside us. In the process, we begin our emergence from the woodenness of life.

Once this process is initiated, as we move outward, we are intended to be taught by what we encounter. Each thing of the world possesses a unique intelligence and soul. Each is always communicating. Those things that we encounter are unique in combination, series, and individuality to us alone. Together they contain meanings meant for ourselves and our life paths alone. They may seem innocuous at first, and only on reflection can we see the meaning in them. From such unremarked events, often unrecognized and unknown, parts of us are awakened, and stirred into life.

We are constantly surrounded by the teachings meant for us. Each of them has a certain odor, a specific shape, that we can come to recognize. We are, after all, meant to recognize them, if only we attend to their presence. We can train ourselves to sense these teachings, learn to follow them with the keenness of perception of a hound lifting his nose at smells wafting over a meadow trail. Learning to track the meanings and communications sent to us as they emerge into our perception is one of the earliest and most essential of spiritual skills. A scholar of indigenous religions, Joseph Epes Brown, speaks of these messages this way.

> The sacred powers may manifest themselves through any form or being of the natural world, which may appear visually, or which may wish to communicate through some audible message. The presence and word of the Great Mystery is within every being, every thing, every event. Even the smallest being, a little ant, for example, may appear and communicate something of the power of the Great Mystery which is behind all forms of creation. The powers and beings of the world wish to communicate with Man; they wish to establish a relationship, but may only do so where the recipient is in a state of humility, and is attentive with all his being.[2]

The immanental world lies deep within this material one; the expressions of the sacred—of deeper meanings—are there for those who wish to see them. The track of the sacred and the teachings that are meant for each of us can be found by those who look for them and learn to perceive them. The capacity for this kind of perception must be cultivated—it is a lifelong training.

The organ of perception for these communications is the heart. It is the heart, as an organ of perception, that is made to sense aisthesis—the soul of the world and the communications that are sent to us. It is this sense that guides us. When we are open to the information that comes from the world through our hearts, we are literally led through the soul-making process that we need to go through to become ourselves.

As we activate the heart's subtle capacity for sophisticated feeling, we free the imprisoned ability of the human to perceive the living reality of things. This allows the unique living essence that is present in all things physically manifested to flow into the human through the organ of perception that is designed to receive it—the heart. The heart has a natural capacity to find the "each-ness" of things, to experience an intimacy with each particular event in a pluralistic cosmos. As we open the heart, the value of each particular thing strikes the heart. We become linked, through the neurological organ whose function it is to perceive in this way, with and to the world. Once we open up and release this formerly frozen capacity, held in captivity by reality-inaccurate modes of thought, the heart becomes, as James Hillman says, an

ardent witness to imaginal persons [that are] independent of the heart which beholds them. Not held; be held, and we beholden to powers; we in their luminosity, watched by them, guarded, remembered, visible presences, en-lightening our darkness by their beauty.[3]

Retreat into the wilderness accompanied by fasting has long been the primary act that frees up the heart as an organ of perception. Once this occurs, the movements of that deeper part of us and the powers that are concerned with our welfare can often be more clearly perceived. Their caring direction for our life can then be seen in the many odd and unique events that have attended us throughout our lives. As the depth of our fasting increases, our awareness of these teachings and of the touch of the sacred also increases. We move in this process from a purely secular life into the deeper life we are meant to live. Our winged self begins to take flight.

Cultivating Sacred Perception and Soul Emergence Through the Fast

When you decide to engage in a transformational fast, there are certain acts that can facilitate the opening of your heart as an organ of perception, your perception of the sacredness of the world, your contact with your deeper self and those powers meant to help you, and your sense of the purpose for which you have been born.

As you enter the wilderness to begin your fast, bring as few things from the material world as possible. Carry instead the intentions you have for the fast. Carry these in the forefront of your mind. During the long days and nights of the fast, as boring or uncomfortable as they might become, keep these things as much as possible in the forefront of your mind. Hold to them with the strength of your desire. And learn to wait.

As the fast progresses, there is often the desire for things to hurry up, to move faster. The desire to skip over all the hard parts of the fast, to get to the cookies on the other side, can become tremendously strong. As much as possible, learn to wait, to calm yourself, to allow yourself to sink down into the experience and observe its movement through your life minute by minute, hour by hour, day by day.

As this process unfolds, allow yourself to think of the reasons why you were born. Begin grappling with the question you have been asked: "What is the purpose of your life?" As you ask yourself this question, notice what feelings arise. Sit with them; do not run off somewhere else, even if only in your mind. You are, after all, asking yourself the most fundamental question of your life. It should not be answered in haste. *Feel* the question; drop down through its layers of meaning. Allow the answer to emerge from your deepest self. Transform your hunger for food into hunger for the answer to this question. Allow your desire to bring the answer back to you. If you truly desire it and wait patiently, the answer will come. Sometimes the powers of the world want to see if you are really serious before they respond.

Think also of the sacred, of the luminous world, of the intelligence and soul that exist in all things. As the veil between you and all other things thins during the progression of the fast, look through it—look for what is waiting for you on the other side. As you work to open yourself to the sacred world, as the first tiny cracks appear, allow it to flow into you, to fill you. As Al-Ghazzali says: "Thus will the reward of the fasting man be generous and even profuse and it will be beyond imagination or estimate."[4] Gandhi says it this way: "No matter from what motive you are fasting, during this precious time, think of your Maker, and of your relation to Him and His other creation, and you will make discoveries you may not have even dreamed of."[5] Walt Whitman puts it succinctly as well: "Be not discouraged, keep on, there are divine things well envelop'd. I swear to you there are divine things more beautiful than words can tell."[6]

As your heart becomes more flexible and your sensitivity to the fluid of communications within which you swim increases, let yourself realize that everything around you, the ground, the stones, the trees, the air, the birds, your blanket—everything—is alive, aware, conscious, intelligent, and speaking to you. For "prayer," as Thomas Merton says, "is not science but poetry." And the poetry of prayer is built on experiencing the invisibles behind all forms of creation and then sending out from the deepest recesses of the human heart communications in return. Human proximity to the invisible world, to the sacred, has never been a matter of location but always one of qualities and attributes. The sacred is everywhere, and although some places—such as wilderness—allow its emergence into human perception more strongly, the core of all things is this sacred ground. So allow yourself to stop, to rest in the moment, to really see. Notice the colors of the things around you. Notice as the fast progresses how these colors deepen, become more alive. Notice what is under these colors, for each thing rightly seen unlocks a new faculty of soul. As your ability to see is enhanced during the fast, feel the meanings in which you are immersed, the meanings that you can perceive with this new way of seeing. This deeper focus is important, for, as Mohammed commented, "many a man gets nothing out of his fast except hunger and thirst." If you concentrate only on the superficial form of things, only the superficial is found. And the most elemental aspect of fasting is hunger and thirst. This hunger and thirst can be used as energy to release the deeper hungers and thirsts that you possess. Direct it outward, *into* the world, and allow yourself to lament, as Black Elk called it. Send your need-questing into the heart of the world with all the power of your hunger behind it, and then notice what comes back to you. The response is often circumspect, the increased sensitivity of your perception necessary to see what is in front of you. The poet Dale Pendell captures this in his poem "Oracles."

> Though the gods have the power of speech
> more often they choose a flower or plant;
> elder leaves pressed on a blotter,
> or spring buds emerging from a winter stem.
>
> These messages they send—
> so ordinary we often miss them:
> an easy laughter and lightness,
> or legs casually crossed and touching,
>
> the way a serpentine dike blends seamlessly into bedrock
> or the way two possible lovers move,
> starting and stopping, passing and pausing
> on an April trail.
>
> The subtlest oracles are always the most obvious—
> seeing what's in front of us the most difficult:
> a butterfly hatching from a ruptured dream,
> or a splintered tree rooting in the soil where it fell—
>
> That those we've left endure or falter
> does not mean that we must also—
> the poison that bit us is also our medicine—
> it is well to name things as they are.
>
> Like that swampy Cree girl they called "Dries
>   Things Out"

when they found her sitting by the stream,
a dragonfly on each palm,
all three drying together in the sun.

The gods' whispers are never commands,
more like the place a steep trail has collapsed,
and sunlight offers the understory
a second chance.[7]

There are communications that are meant for you that come from the heart of the world, from the powers that are here to help you, from the soul that is within everything around you. These communications are a food that is more filling than bread, more nutrient-rich than the greenest leaf, more energy-loaded than sugar, more strength-giving than meat, and headier than wine.

You may become aware of a tremendous loneliness from your movement away from food, television, newspapers, friends, relatives, work, your daily culture. Often these feelings of loneliness are hidden behind or underneath the noisiness of daily life. Binge eating or overeating can also be a way to stuff these feelings down, to keep them away, to avoid the pain of their expression. Fasting brings you face-to-face with this loneliness. For during a deep wilderness fast there is nothing but you, the place of your retreat, and the immeasurably vast Universe around you. Don't run from these feelings but sit with them and allow yourself to sink down into them. Look out at the world from this place, this deep loneliness. These "emotions of bleakness," as Hillman comments, "are the reactions of the heart to the anesthetic life in our civilization."[8] And this bleakness is not unique to our time but concomitant to a life submerged in the superficial—something that happens to every human being in every age in every culture. It is a desert that resides within every human heart; such loneliness is an archetypal experience of the human being. It is neither a sin, nor a condition, nor a disease, not abnormal, nor unusual. Such loneliness is essential to the human being, for its presence points the way that each of us must go.

The solution to this bleakness, this powerful loneliness, is not in suppressing it or in running from it but in facing it, in going through it to the other side. All of us struggle with the predicament of the human condition; all of us must face this loneliness, this desert within us. Historically, one way to work with it, to go through it, to come to terms with it, is to travel into the actual desert and to fast. When we stay for an extended period in the desert, we must face the desert within our own hearts. We are forced to look at its terrain, to walk its landscape, to seek springs that humans in long times past once knew and drank from. Without the hunger and thirst that come from voluntarily abstaining from food, often there is neither sufficient motivation to find those springs nor the incomparable joy of drinking from them.

Encountering this loneliness, this bleakness, can feel tremendously debilitating at first. As time progresses, something begins to awaken in us in response—strong passions, often rage. This is important, for, as Hillman comments, "the passions of the soul make the desert habitable."[9] It is only the power of our passion that can take us through the difficulty of this loneliness. When we allow these strong passions to emerge within us and begin to direct them, to own their power, something within us is healed. Becoming angry is crucial in this coming-to-terms. It is essential to becoming whole.

Encountering this archetypal loneliness of the human spirit leads directly into another element of deep fasting—thinking back over your life. The deep fast is a time of coming to terms as well as finding new, and better, food. It is almost always true that during deep wilderness fasting people have a tendency to ruminate on their failings, sometimes to feel that their unkindnesses are too many, that they are not holy enough, or pure enough, or lovable enough to find forgiveness or find a deeper spiritual life. This is not so. Take the risk to quest with the heart and mind you actually have, not with the mind and heart you think you are supposed to have. If you allow these things that trouble you to simply *be* and ask earnestly with all your heart for help, then help you will surely find. For all of us are only human beings. All of us have failed, all of us have been unkind, all of us have betrayed, and have been betrayed. It is an inescapable part of the journey. What matters is what you do with it now. It is a great act of intimacy to show yourself and the Universe the parts of yourself that you feel are unworthy. Many people believe that by exposing these vulnerabilities so plainly, they risk losing the love of God. For why will the sacred *not* turn away from you, once you are stripped bare, as others you have loved have done? This is one of the most powerful healing acts of any deep wilderness fast. It is only when we risk this most basic and soul-challenging vulnerability that we can find that truly we are loved for what we are and who we are and needed for what we bring. We are in fact wanted.

During this reflection on your life, notice the patterns that have been present throughout your life; the opportunities that you were given that seemingly came from nowhere; the odd ways the Universe sometimes seemed to open up to you and bring you the things you needed. Notice the patterns of your successes and how magical everything has sometimes seemed. Notice also the patterns of your failures. There are times for each of us when nothing we do seems to work well, when everything has some strange failure in it. What was the deeper message in these failures? What was it that you did not want to hear? These periods of failure can often be great teachers for us. There is often a deep wisdom in such patterns of failure that, if understood and owned, can lead the way to an increased maturity and strength of character.

This focused reflection on the deeper meanings in the events of our lives is essential. As Thomas Merton teaches: "All our journeys begin as human journeys. It is only later that they become consciously spiritual. Our origins often hold the key to our future and form the core of our spirituality."[10]

The fast is above all a means for becoming conscious. Becoming conscious entails coming to terms with those things that have been unconscious. It means coming out of denial. It means reclaiming an intimacy with yourself that, perhaps, you have not known in years. It also means becoming intimate with the soul that resides in the world. To do so means exposing, and allowing the fast to heal, your deepest heart. This personal intimacy allows you to live from the deepest part of yourself outward, for no longer do you need to cover this deep self or ignore its communications. As the writer Audre Lorde comments, this makes a tremendous difference in *how* life is experienced.

> When we begin to live from within outward, in touch with the power of the erotic within ourselves, then we begin to be responsible to ourselves in the deepest sense. For as we recognize our deepest feelings, we begin to give up, of necessity, being satisfied with suffering and self-negation, and the numbness which so often seems the only alternative in our society."[11]

During the process of exploring these many experiences, you may experience a great many feelings. It is not uncommon for people to experience deep grief during wilderness fasts. The grief that is released during such times has been there for a long time. When you allow yourself to express it, held in the arms of the world, cushioned by the hands of the Earth, you give yourself one of the greatest gifts you can offer. It is an act of incredible compassion and love.

The dams that are built on the rivers of the world have their counterparts in each of us. We are often taught in the West that we must not cry, especially if we are men. But such dams can be removed. The freshness and release of energy that comes from this act is indescribably sweet and powerful. This alone is enough to alter the fabric of normal, everyday life. It takes a lot of energy to hold such grief at bay; releasing the grief back into the world frees up *all* the energy formerly needed to repress it.

When you respond to your deepest self with compassion and kindness and do not punish yourself afterward—when, as Geneen Roth comments, "you experience even the palest glimmer of self-love, it becomes increasingly difficult to feel comfortable in relationships where all that exists is the pretense of love."[12]

The fast can offer much more than food deprivation, much more than healing for the body. It also offers the deepest kind of healing for the soul within you. When you accept the challenge of traveling into the wilderness within yourself, you begin to fight for the life of the soul. The bounty you receive is, as Robert Bly commented, "not fame, not wages, not friends, but what is already in the soul, a freshness that no one can destroy."

Appendix 1:

A 10-Week, Low-Fat Cleansing Diet

The following diet is exceptionally good for preparing your body, mind, and spirit for a fast. Spending some time on this kind of diet will allow your body to gradually adjust to the changes that it is going to be experiencing.

1. Drink 4–6 glasses of water every day. Do not use tap water.
2. Eliminate dairy products, eggs, and sweets.
3. Eat only *whole* grains (brown rice, millet, barley, oats, quinoa, and so on), organic beans, lightly steamed organic vegetables and fruits, and minimal wild or free-range meats. Tempeh and tofu are excellent. *Do not cook any grains with oil.*
4. Use only olive oil for cooking. Use no more than 2 tablespoons of oil per day. Do not use butter or margarine of any kind.
5. Drink all the fresh vegetable and fruit juices you like.
6. Do not use salt. Any other spices you wish are okay, as are small amounts of tamari and soy.
7. Do not use any caffeinated drinks (except green tea), alcohol, or recreational drugs during the diet. If you

are a heavy caffeine drinker, instead of stopping cold turkey, go from coffee to black tea to green tea over a 1- to 2-week period of time.

8. Eat fruits first and alone. They digest rapidly and when eaten with other foods are held in the stomach, where they can cause gas and intestinal upset.

9. Do not eat any fried foods.

10. Consider consuming a "green drink" each morning. Many of these are powdered and must be mixed into juice and blended. A Fresh Green Drink is described in appendix 2.

FOOD LIST

Buy only organic, pesticide-free foods. This is important. The chemicals in nonorganically farmed foods will be taken into the body where they can have powerful impacts. You are working to lessen your toxin load; organic foods remove one common source of toxins that are often hard for the liver to process. This takes the load off the liver and allows it to work more efficiently in helping your body detoxify.

Fruits: Use any fruits you wish.

Vegetables:

artichoke	swiss chard	snow peas	zucchini
collards	daikon greens	burdock	broccoli
corn	string beans	beets	cucumber
acorn squash	watercress	onion	daikon
turnip greens	red radish	kale	jicama
spinach	asparagus	mustard	celery
cabbage	cauliflower	greens	raw carrots

all sprouts	parsnips	summer squash	potatoes, red or white
romaine	cooked carrots		
butternut squash	brussels sprouts	rutabagas	turnips
		red leaf lettuce	avocados
pumpkins	sweet potatoes		
tomatoes	parsley	eggplant	

Oil: Use olive oil for cooking. Flaxseed oil, because of its high levels of omega-3 oils, is a very good oil to use (uncooked) for such things as salad dressings.

Salad Dressings: Use herbed vinegar, champagne, wine, or fruit vinegars only—combine with flaxseed oil if desired.

Seasonings: Any are okay except salt.

Beverages:
- Water: Filtered or artisan spring water. Do not use distilled water. Avoid all frozen concentrated juices.
- Herbal teas: Especially ginger, peppermint, and chamomile.

Meats: Fish from the sea, especially cold-water fish. If you feel you want fowl, use only range-fed, pharmaceutical-free, organic chickens (or other birds). Wild meats such as venison or elk are excellent; if they are farmed, they should be organic. Meat should be eaten only once or twice a week during the diet. *Note:* Salmon is almost always raised in pens in the sea. These fish are highly dosed with growth stimulants, food colorings, and antibiotics. They should be avoided. Eat only wild sea salmon. (Catfish is also farm raised.)

Breads: Use only sprouted grain breads.

Cooking: Use only stainless steel, enameled, or earthenware cooking utensils. Never use aluminum.

Sweeteners: Use pure maple syrup. Maple syrup contains enough essential ingredients that it is possible to live on it for extended periods of time. It supplies nearly all the essential vitamins and minerals necessary for health.

GUIDELINES

It is best to establish a routine for meals and a list of meals *before* you start on the diet. Cook a large pot of grain of your choice and keep it in the refrigerator. This way if you get hungry there is already something available.

Eat as much as you wish throughout the day. Fruit is good as a snack food. Have it available to eat whenever you feel hungry. It is helpful to get a good vegetarian cookbook and plan out a week's meals.

SAMPLE DAILY MENUS

- *Breakfast:* (1) Herbal tea, oatmeal with raisins and maple syrup. (2) Fruit salad. (3) Powdered or Fresh Green Drink.
- *Lunch:* Vegetable soup, sprouted bread, or rice and steamed vegetables with tamari.
- *Dinner:* (1) Steamed vegetables or vegetable casserole, grain of choice, salad with herbed vinegar. (2) Steamed salmon with dill and lime; steamed asparagus; wild green salad with snow peas and radish.

POWDERED GREEN DRINKS

"Green drinks" have become more popular of late, and a number of types are readily available in health food stores and on the Internet. You can buy them premixed (follow the directions on the container) or make them yourself. The one I make contains

2 parts each of spirulina, Siberian ginseng, nettle leaf, astragalus, tumeric, dandelion root, and milk thistle seed and 1 part each of chlorella, bladderwrack (a seaweed), burdock, and ashwaghanda. I add ⅓ cup of the powdered mixture to 12 ounces of apple juice and 1 tablespoon of flaxseed oil and blend, then drink. It is more effective if you begin blending the apple juice first, then add the oil and powdered herbs. Otherwise it clumps. This drink is just about as healthy a thing as you can take, and it is very filling, especially if taken at breakfast.

THINGS TO REMEMBER

1. It is normal to feel a sensation that is usually described as hunger no matter how much you eat in the early days (up to 2 weeks) of this kind of diet. It is not actually hunger but the shift away from a high carbohydrate/glucose diet. During this time your body will begin using more fat stores, shifting partially into ketosis, to make up the calorie difference. By the end of the diet most people generally feel increased energy, have more mental alertness and little hunger, eat smaller portions, are highly relaxed, and have lower stress levels.
2. You may feel lightheaded; this is also normal.
3. Since eating is such a social event, it is normal to feel left out when others go out to eat. Go with them and convince them to go to a good health food restaurant. Order food that comes from this list and is light on oils.
4. When others order alcohol and you also wish to drink, order sparkling water with a lime in a champagne glass.

5. Emotional issues often arise during any change in eating patterns, especially when the body is using up its stores of fat. Remember that this is normal and make no major life decisions during this time. Remember: this, too, shall pass.

Appendix 2:

Juices for Fasting

My favorite combinations for juice fasting or preparing my body for water fasting are the recipes I offer here for the Detox Blend, the Fresh Green Drink, the Cleansing Blend 1, or the Cleansing Blend 2. There are a great many possible juice blends that can be used for fasting—these are only four possibilities. The two best overall sources for information on juicing, juice combinations, and the health benefits of different juices are John Heinerman, *Heinerman's Encyclopedia of Healing Juices,* and Michael Murray, *The Complete Book of Juicing.*

I, like many people who came of age in the 1960s, use a Champion juicer, the workhorse of juicers. It is extremely durable and relatively inexpensive. Its primary limitation is that it cannot juice wheatgrass, which needs a special type of machine. It is possible to buy juicers that do both wheatgrass and pretty much everything else—even such exotic items as pine needles. These are more expensive. The best way to find a juicer is to do a comparison search on the Internet—try www.google.com. There are sites that specialize in juicers, and they often offer extremely low prices.

As always, you should try to buy only organic vegetables and herbs for juicing. Not only will this avoid as much chemical contamination as possible but the mineral and vitamin content of organic foods is much higher. Over the past 40 years the mineral content of most vegetables has declined between 25 and 35 percent because of the way they are grown. The nutritional information that follows is based on averages for organic vegetables.

DETOX BLEND

This blend is the best juice combination I have found for supporting and enhancing the detoxification of the body. It strongly supports liver and kidney function—helps them work more efficiently, optimizes their ability to cleanse the body of built-up toxins, and helps them heal and regenerate. If you are not used to the potency of beets, start slow with the size of the beets you use and work up. They can be exceptionally strong in their effects.

Detox Blend

5–7 carrots
3–4 fresh celery stalks
1 small or medium beet
(optional: ½ apple)

Juice and drink, 1–3 times daily.

My first experience with a large beet (no, I did not start out small and work up—I'm a guy) was about like drinking a couple of espressos in quick succession, at least in terms of the energy rush. I also felt slightly faint and slightly nauseous and spent a lot of time in the bathroom—beets stimulate bowel movements. Because the urine and feces were reddish in color, I was convinced I was bleeding internally. The headline was stark in my mine: *Local Man Dies from Health Food Diet Fad*.

Beets do that to people.

ABOUT THE INGREDIENTS

Beet (*Beta vulgaris*)

One medium beet (without tops) contains approximately: 250 mg potassium, 50 mg sodium, 10 mg calcium, 35 mg phosphorus, 0.5 mg iron, 20 International Units (I.U.) vitamin A, 75 mcg folic acid, 8 mg vitamin C, and trace amounts of the B vitamins thiamine, riboflavin, niacin, and B-6. Beets contain betaine (also found in milk thistle seed), the amino acids asparagine and glutamine, a number of fruit acids, sugar compounds, and triterpene saponins. Beets (and their compound betaine) are a strong liver protector and liver regenerator. They are also a strong cholagogue, stimulating bile production and flow. Some physicians in Europe commonly use beets, quite successfully, as a primary treatment for hepatitis. (They have also been used for cancer, alcoholism, and venous insufficiency.) Beets are one of the most powerful of the liver-detoxifying plants and as such have a primary place in any detoxification program. They flush the liver quite rapidly and supply a strong energy surge at the same time. The betaine in beets is essential to the detoxification processes of the liver, especially those that work through methylation. Methylation is used by the body to detoxify the natural, body-produced compounds dopamine, epinephrine (adrenaline from the adrenal glands), histamines, and a number of different types of pharmaceuticals.

If you are not used to them, beets should be used in moderation; 1 small beet per glass of juice. Once you are accustomed to them, use 1 medium beet.

> *Warning:* Beet juice is extremely strong in its effects and should be mixed with other juices. Do not use with obstructed bile duct.

NOTE: Beet juice will turn both urine and stool reddish. What you see is not blood.

Celery (*Apium graveolens*)

Two stalks of celery contain (approximately) the following nutrients: 275 mg potassium, 30 mg magnesium, 35 mg calcium, 20 mg phosphorus, 90 mg sodium, 225 I.U. vitamin A, 8 mg vitamin C, 0.2 mg iron, 8 mcg folic acid, and trace amounts of thiamine, riboflavin, niacin, and B-6.

Celery is closely related to a number of very powerful medicinal plants: osha (*Ligusticum porterii*), angelica (*Angelica archangelica*), and lomatium (*Lomatium dissectum*). It is not surprising that celery also possesses a number of very powerful medicinal actions. Like these other plants, celery is antimicrobial, antibacterial, slightly antiviral, antispasmodic, and anti-inflammatory.

Celery is especially useful for lowering blood pressure. It contains a compound, 3-n-butyl phthalide, which can lower blood pressure about 14 percent when taken in sufficient quantities. It is also high in apigenin, a blood vessel dilator, which also helps lower blood pressure. Three to four celery stalks will supply the necessary amount of both compounds to lower blood pressure. Celery also contains a large number of compounds that act like calcium-channel blockers and that help reduce and prevent angina. The apigenin, magnesium, potassium, and another compound, apiin, in celery make it a useful herb as well for cardiac arrhythmia. In a number of studies, celery juice has also been found to significantly reduce cholesterol levels in the blood. Celery is a strong antioxidant and is also reliably effective in lowering the levels of uric acid in the body by stimulating its excretion in the urine. Historically, this has made it a primary remedy for gout. Normally the seeds are used, but the fresh plant juice, while slightly weaker in action, produces the same result. Celery has also been found effective for helping to alleviate arthritis and rheumatic complaints, skin rashes and diseases, nervousness (especially accompanied by anxiety), upset stomach and digestive system, and gallstones.

But celery's major areas of importance for fasting are its impacts on the kidneys. Its wide-ranging impacts on kidney function help the removal of toxins from the body through the kidneys by enhancing kidney function and urine flow. Because part of the primary function of the kidneys is to filter the blood and maintain the body's electrolyte balance, the use of celery during juice fasting supports optimum filtration and electrolyte balances. Electrolyte balance is also enhanced by the large amounts of primary electrolytes—calcium, magnesium, and potassium—in celery.

Celery is a specific remedy for the kidneys. It is a kidney tonic and an antimicrobial, antispasmodic, and anti-inflammatory for the urinary passages; reduces kidney stone formation; increases urine flow (a diuretic); and (in Chinese medicine) helps alleviate dizziness. Celery's volatile oil, apiol, is excreted through the urinary tract and acts as a mild but reliable urinary system antiseptic.

Researchers have also found a male steroid in celery. The chemical (5 *alpha*-androst-16-en-3 *alpha*-ol) and its related, 3-ketone, combine together to form the chemicals that in a number of animals stimulate sexual arousal in the female; they are a sign of elevated sex hormones in the male and its readiness to mate. The two compounds are closely related in structure to both androstene-dione and testosterone. They are present in these vegetables at about the level of 8 ng/gm of fresh weight, a moderately high level, and perhaps explain why celery has long been used as a sexual tonic for men.

In short, celery affects the entire urinary network and most of the bodily systems that the kidneys affect: heart, digestive system, adrenals, and blood vessels.

Suggested dosage: Three to four celery stalks juiced daily (makes 3–4 ounces of juice).

> *Warning:* Fresh celery juice, taken in quantity, will cause a slight numbing of the tongue. Large doses of celery juice are contraindicated in kidney disease. The roots will sometimes, because of improper storage, become infected with yeasts that can raise the furocumarin content of the roots by 200 percent. These furocumarin-enhanced roots can cause phototoxicosis. Use only fresh celery. In rare circumstances celery can cause allergic reactions, or even anaphylactic shock in some individuals. Do not use if you have a history of allergic reaction.

Carrot (*Daucus carota*)

Five medium carrots contain somewhere in the range of: 125 mg calcium, 1,250 mg potassium, 40 mg magnesium, 125 mg phosphorus, 170 mg sodium, 40,000 I.U. vitamin A, 30 mg vitamin C, 2.5 mg iron, 50 mcg folic acid, and trace amounts of thiamine, riboflavin, niacin, and B-6.

Carrots are a member of the same family as celery and possess many of the same actions. They are exceptionally good for angina, high blood pressure, and high cholesterol levels. The seeds and stems are stronger in these actions, though the root is active as well. But two actions of carrot roots merit particular attention: those actions that are generated by the various carotenoids in carrot roots and their impacts on the liver.

Carrot roots are extremely high in carotenoids (including beta-carotene). These are the compounds that give carrots their orange color. Researchers at the pharmaceutical giant Hoffmann–La Roche cite more than 30 studies showing that carotenoids help prevent the three Cs: cancer, cardiovascular disease, and cataracts. (They are also especially good in helping prevent stroke.) A decade-long Harvard study showed that 50 mg of carotenoids *every other day* significantly reduces the risks of these three diseases. It takes the juice of about 7 carrots to produce 50 mg. (Five carrots will produce about 35 mg.) Research on carotenes is showing that they possess a wide range of action in the human body. Beta-carotene is considered to be a provitamin, that is, the body turns it into vitamin A. A number of carotenes have been found to have significant antioxidant activity. They protect the thymus gland and enhance its functioning and have strong immune-enhancing effects. Studies show that 180 mg a day of beta-carotene (300,000 I.U.) increases the number of helper/inducer T-cells of the immune system by 30 percent after 7 days and all T-cells after 14 days. Studies have found that even 15 mg per day of beta-carotene significantly improves immune function. However, if those 15 mg come from the ingestion of carrots rather than a synthetic supplement, immune enhancement is much greater.

Carotenes also appear to increase the structural integrity of the cellular lining of the respiratory tract and decrease leukotriene formation. This makes them useful in the treatment and prevention of asthma and other allergic respiratory responses. They are also extremely effective in maintaining and restoring healthy eye function.

The central portion of the macula of the eye is yellow in color, mainly from the presence of two yellow carotenes: lutein and zeaxanthin. Carrots improve eye function in part because their carotenes are strongly supportive of the macula and can even help prevent macular degeneration when used regularly. The beta-carotenes from carrots can also help prevent cataracts and improve night vision.

Carotenoids also are extremely useful in the treatment of skin diseases. They tend to decrease wrinkling from aging of the skin and are sometimes highly effective in the treatment of acne.

The liver-enhancing effects of carrots are not as well known as their effects on the eyes and those that come from their carotenoids. However, carrots have been used for a long time in India in the treatment of liver diseases. Recent research there has

Warning: There is one instance of a young man ingesting such significant quantities of pure carrot juice (the amounts were never specified but apparently were very large) that he caused cirrhosis of the liver. Vitamin A in large quantities can cause liver damage and is quite toxic in overdose. That supplied from foods is much less toxic, though extreme amounts can be damaging. Large amounts of carrot juice are contraindicated for people with active liver disease.

shown that carrots can provide significant protection for the liver from chemical pollutants. A number of compounds in carrots increase the activity of several enzymes that enhance the detoxification actions of the liver, and some evidence exists that carrots can help remove heavy metal contaminants from the body as well.

Suggested dosage: 5–7 juiced medium carrots per glass of juice.

Apple (*Pyrus malus*)

One-half of an unpeeled apple contains 4 mg vitamin C, 80 mg potassium, 7 I.U. vitamin A, 5 mg calcium, 3 mg magnesium, 5 mg phosphorus, and traces of chromium, thiamine, riboflavin, niacin, sodium, and iron. Some of the more important contents of unpeeled apples are: carotenoids, pectin, ellagic acid, chlorogenic acid, and caffeic acid.

Pectin is a gel-forming compound that is most often used in jams and jellies to make them gel. It also helps form a gel within the intestinal tract, facilitating the intestines' ability to move fecal matter through the bowels. This is one of the things that makes apples, apple juice, and apple sauce so good for constipation. Pectin also binds to and helps eliminate toxins in the bowels.

Ellagic acid protects chromosomes from damage and exerts strong protective actions against many pollutants' tendency to damage DNA. Studies have shown that ellagic acid blocks the action of numerous cancer-causing agents, among them the collective compounds in cigarette smoke known as polycyclic aromatic hydrocarbons. Ellagic acid is a powerful antioxidant and acts in the body to increase other antioxidant compounds including the potent molecular compound glutathione. Glutathione is perhaps one of the most powerful antioxidants in the body.

Dosage: ½ juiced apple added to juice blend per day if desired.

FRESH GREEN DRINK

A fresh green drink is especially good if you intend a lengthy juice fast. Green vegetables contain a number of powerful actions and nutrients that celery, by itself, and root vegetables do not have. This is a particularly refreshing blend.

Fresh Green Drink

2 fresh celery stalks
½ cucumber
1 large fresh kale leaf
½ cup fresh spinach
small sprig parsley to taste
1 ounce wheatgrass juice (if available)
(optional: 1–3 radishes)

ABOUT THE INGREDIENTS

Cucumber (*Cucumis sativus*)

One-half an average cucumber contains 260 I.U. vitamin A, 220 mg potassium, 20 mcg folic acid, 20 mg calcium, 15 mg magnesium, 25 mg phosphorus, 5 mg sodium, moderate amounts of silica and chlorophyll, and trace amounts of vitamin C, thiamine, riboflavin, niacin, B-6, boron, and iron.

Cucumbers are a mild diuretic; their seeds cause mild tonic actions on the kidneys, help prevent kidney stones, and promote uric acid excretion from the body. Cucumbers, especially the peel, are exceptionally good for promoting healthy skin, keeping it elastic and reducing wrinkles. I like cucumbers in green drinks because they contribute a *lot* of water, diluting the intensity of the other plants in the mixture.

Suggested dosage: ½ cucumber per green drink.

NOTE: Do not peel cucumbers but juice them whole.

Kale (*Brassica oleracea*)
Kale is especially high in beneficial nutrients such as carotenes (see carrots) and chlorophyll. One large kale leaf with stem (about 3 ounces) contains 10,000 I.U. vitamin A, 100 mg vitamin C, 175 mcg folic acid, 250 mg potassium, 200 mg calcium, 2 mg iron, 15 mg magnesium, 60 mg phosphorus, 3 mg sodium, 2 mg niacin, and trace amounts of thiamine, riboflavin, B-6, copper, manganese, and zinc.

A cup of kale or collard greens has more calcium than a glass of milk and is much better assimilated in this form into the body. Kale, like other members of the brassica family (such as cabbage, broccoli, and cauliflower) possesses potent anticancer compounds and a rich supply of antioxidants.

Suggested dosage: 1 large leaf with stem per green drink.

Spinach (*Spinacea oleracea*)
Like other dark green leafy vegetables, spinach contains large amounts of chlorophyll and carotenes—all of which are potent cancer protectors. One cup of fresh, raw spinach contains 3,750 I.U. vitamin A, 16 mg vitamin C, 110 mcg folic acid, 300 mg potassium, 60 mg calcium, 1.5 mg iron, 45 mg magnesium, 30 mg phosphorus, 22 mg sodium, and trace amounts of thiamine, riboflavin, niacin, and B-6.

Suggested dosage: ½ cup fresh spinach.

Parsley (*Petroselinum crispum*)
Parsley is a member of the same family as carrots and celery. It is exceptionally high in its chlorophyll content and possesses significant amounts of various carotenes and flavonoids. One-half cup of

parsley contains 1,500 I.U. vitamin A, 25 mg vitamin C, 55 mcg folic acid, 160 mg potassium, 40 mg calcium, 2 mg iron, 15 mg magnesium, 12 mg phosphorus, 12 mg sodium, and trace amounts of niacin, thiamine, riboflavin, and B-6.

Suggested dosage: To taste. Parsley is *very* strong in flavor and takes some getting used to. Start with one small sprig and work up.

Wheatgrass (*Triticum* spp.)
One ounce of fresh wheatgrass juice is 70 percent chlorophyll. It also contains approximately 2,000 I.U. vitamin A, 350 mcg vitamin K, 15 mg vitamin C, 10 mcg thiamine, 1 mg choline, 70 mcg riboflavin, 45 mcg pyroxidine, 1 mcg B-12, 265 mcg niacin, 84 mcg pantothenic acid, 4 mcg biotin, 38 mcg folic acid, 54 mcg boron, 15 mg calcium, 2 mcg chromium, 25 mcg copper, 11 mg magnesium, 12 mcg molybdenum, 22 mg phosphorus, 275 mg potassium, 310 mcg selenium, 940 mcg silicon, 3 mcg vanadium, and traces of iron, manganese, sodium, zinc, and germanium. Wheatgrass juice contains a great many amino acids, including lysine, tryptophan, phenylalanine, isoleucine, leucine, methionine, proline, threonine, valine, alanine, arginine, aspartic acid, glutamine, glycine, histidine, serine, and tyrosine. It is also high in the powerful antioxidant superoxide dismutase (SOD).

A great many claims are made about wheatgrass juice, pretty much that it can cure everything. Ann Wigamore in Boston did the most to popularize its use, and her clinical work in curing thousands of people is the basis of many of the claims for this herb's effectiveness. There have been few clinical studies. However, it is a significant source of a great many beneficial substances and thus helps to counteract chronic low intake of many essential amino acids, vitamins, and minerals. It also appears to help promote the detoxification systems of the liver, lymph system, and kidneys. The ingestion of wheatgrass juice does produce a strong energy surge about 20 minutes after consumption.

Dosage: 1 ounce fresh or fresh-frozen wheatgrass juice added to green drink.

NOTE: Amounts larger than 1 ounce in those unused to its effects can cause nausea.

Radish (*Raphanus sativus*)

There are a number of different types of radishes; all can be used and are of benefit. The most commonly known is the red, but there is a Japanese radish, the daikon, that looks something like a white carrot. There are also black radishes; used mostly in Russia and the eastern European countries, they look much like a very black beet, although inside they possess the normal crisp, white flesh of a radish. All three taste much the same. Daikon radishes are always available in Oriental markets and sometimes in health food stores. Black radishes can mostly be found in neighborhood markets that have large numbers of Russian or Polish customers.

A single medium-sized red radish contains in the neighborhood of 25 mg potassium, 2.5 mg each calcium and phosphorus, 1.5 mg sodium, 1 I.U. of vitamin A, 2 mg vitamin C, and varying traces of magnesium, selenium, iron, and zinc.

Radishes tend to normalize the production of T4, or thyroxine, in the thyroid gland. If too much T4 is being produced, radishes bring levels up; if too little, they lower them. They are in fact a thyroid tonic herb and can be very helpful in treating thyroid problems. Radishes contain a unique compound, raphinin, which normalizes not only thyroxine but also calcitonin, another hormone produced in the thyroid gland. Thyroid-produced calcitonin controls the amount of calcium released into the blood and affects the amount of calcium laid down in the bones during bone matrix formation. With regular intake of radishes or radish juice, the thyroid production of these compounds are normalized. Russian physicians have successfully used radishes for decades for alleviating both hyperthyroidism and hypothyroidism.

Radishes have been found in a number of clinical studies in Malaysia to be powerful inhibitors of kidney stones in prior sufferers who consume them regularly. They also help the liver work with fat intake in the diet more effectively, seem to help break up fat deposits in fatty liver conditions, and help break up gallstones in the gall bladder.

Dosage: If desired, 1–3 medium red radishes, juiced, or the equivalent amount of juiced daikon or black radish. They are spicy, as you know, so start with one and then use more if you like it.

CLEANSING BLENDS I AND 2

These two cleansing blends differ in their energetics. The first one is strongly energetic and stimulating; the second is more tonic, nutritive, and gently supportive. The first one is best used only on a short-term basis for fasts up to 10 days in length; the second is great for both short-term and longer fasts of 10–45 days. The first blend (which is also very good for colds and the flu) is especially good for stimulating the circulatory system. This helps support both the liver and kidneys in detoxifying the body. The second blend, often known as the Master Cleanser Diet (created by Stanley Burroughs), is a very good choice if you have not fasted before. It will give you enough energy to work and carry out daily tasks, most or all necessary bodily nutrients are provided, and it is very

Cleansing Blend 1

10 ounces spring water, hot
4–5 ounces fresh ginger root
¼ fresh lime, squeezed into drink
1 tablespoon organic wildflower honey
⅟₁₆–⅛ teaspoon cayenne

Add juiced ginger, squeezed lime and its juice, honey, and cayenne to hot water. Drink 3–6 times daily, more if desired.

Cleansing Blend 2:
The Master Cleanser Diet

10 ounces spring water, medium hot
2 tablespoons fresh lime or lemon juice
2 tablespoons pure organic maple syrup
⅟₁₆–⅛ teaspoon cayenne

Add squeezed lime or lemon and its juice, maple syrup, and cayenne to hot water. Drink 6–12 glasses daily, more if desired.

easy to make and use—there is no need for juicing at all. Some people simply fill a nipple-fitted, quart-size water bottle and carry it with them all day, drinking the blend whenever desired.

NOTE: Do not substitute honey for maple syrup in Cleansing Blend 2.

ABOUT THE INGREDIENTS

Ginger (*Zingiber officinale*)

Ginger is considered more of a medicinal herb or a spice, not so much a source of nutrients. However, it does possess about 1 percent by weight of calcium, phosphorus, and iron. It is somewhat high in the B vitamins, particularly thiamine, riboflavin, and niacin. It also contains a fair amount of vitamin C.

Ginger is foremost a circulatory herb that has pronounced effects on the heart and blood. Ginger causes the blood vessels to relax and expand, lowering blood pressure and allowing the heart to beat more slowly to pump the blood throughout the body. This, combined with a ginger-stimulated stronger beat of the heart, means that the blood is pumped more efficiently throughout the body. Japanese researchers have found that blood pressure typically lowers 10–15 percent after ingesting ginger. Indian researchers have found that ginger is effective in lowering the cholesterol content of the blood. Dutch researchers have noted it to be efficient in preventing the blood from clotting—similar in its effectiveness to aspirin. Ginger also soothes the stomach, helping indigestion and stimulating healthy digestion. It relieves gas or flatulence and cramping and facilitates absorption of foods in the stomach. A number of researchers have found that ginger is highly effective in alleviating motion sickness, nausea, and vomiting, being more effective than Dramamine, the usual drug of choice for those conditions. It has also been shown to be quite effective for morning sickness. Numerous studies have shown that ginger alleviates the symptoms of arthritis.

Ginger is a potent inhibitor of the inflammatory compounds known as prostaglandins and thromboxanes, which is one of the reasons why it so powerfully helps alleviate arthritic conditions. It is also a strong antioxidant and contains a protein-digesting enzyme (a protease) that appears to have strong impacts on inflammatory processes in the body.

Ginger is strongly antibacterial, with potent activity against a number of human pathogenic bacteria, as well as the foodborne bacteria *Shigella, E. coli,* and *Salmonella.* Its antitussive (anticough) action rivals that of codeine, and it is a strong expectorant that helps move bronchial mucus up and out of the system.

Suggested dosage: Start with a piece about the size of your thumb and work up. You can either grate the fresh ginger and then steep it in the hot water for 20–30 minutes or juice it in a juicer and simply add the juice to the hot water. I usually juice it.

Many people start with about 1 ounce of juice and then increase the amount of juiced ginger as desired and as they become used to it. I prefer 4–5 ounces at this point, but I really like the spicy flavor, and I really enjoy the effects of ginger on my metabolism. I also save the juiced pulp and steep it in 10 ounces of hot water for a second cup later in the day. I find this to be as strong a tea as that from the original juice.

Lime *(Citrus aurantifolia)* or Lemon *(Citrus lemon)*
One-quarter of a lime contains 4 mg calcium, 20 mg potassium, 2 mg phosphorus, 5 mg vitamin C, 0.25 mg sodium, 1 mg magnesium, and varying trace amounts of iron, A and B-complex vitamins, germanium, tin, selenium, and zinc. Lemon is a bit higher in most of these, mostly due to its larger size. Lime (and lemon as well) is strongly antibacterial and antimicrobial. It also contains (especially the peel) flavonoids, including rutin. These compounds affect vascular permeability; essentially, they strengthen the walls of capillaries and blood vessels. This helps reduce vari-

cose veins, for instance, and plays a role in preventing stroke and hemorrhoids. Limes are mildly anti-inflammatory and diuretic; they help increase urine production and expression. Limes (and lemons) also contain limonene, which, while it helps dissolve gallstones, is showing great promise in both preventing and treating cancer. It strongly enhances the action of detoxification enzymes in the liver. This not only is effective in helping treat and prevent cancer but is especially good for helping enhance the liver's ability to process the body's accumulated toxins. Limonene is specifically necessary for the parts of the liver's detoxification system that work through glutathione conjugation and glucuronidation. These two processes deactivate acetaminophen, nicotine, organophosphates (insecticides), various carcinogens, and a number of pharmaceuticals.

Limonene is mostly present in the white, spongy inner pith—between the peel and the inner fruit—of limes and lemons. Because the peel and pith are so biologically active, it is more beneficial to squeeze the lime or lemon wedge into the drink and then drop it in as well and let it steep.

Suggested dosage: ¼ fresh lime squeezed into glass and dropped into glass as well. Lemon can be used interchangeably, I just like the taste of lime better in Cleansing Blend 1.

Cayenne (*Capsicum minimum*)

Cayenne is extremely high in vitamin C, copper, and phosphorus; is high in vitamin A; and is a good source of bioflavonoids, potassium, and vitamin E.

Cayenne increases the body's metabolic rate—in some studies by as much as 25 percent. This causes the body to burn more fat as fuel and makes cayenne especially helpful in increasing weight loss when taken during fasting. Cayenne also increases blood circulation, dilates capillaries, increases blood flow to outlying portions of the body, and lowers blood pressure. These actions make it especially useful during cleansing fasts. Cayenne is also a potent pain reliever. It contains capsaicin, a compound that stimulates the release of endorphins, the body's natural pain relievers. A number of studies have found it to be exceptionally effective in the treatment of cluster headaches and the pain of arthritis. Cayenne is also a powerful antiseptic and breaks up mucus throughout the respiratory tract and helps it move up and out of the system.

Because fasting can sometimes be accompanied by pain (joint or headaches) and is almost always accompanied by coldness in the extremities, cayenne, besides its powerful actions on the circulatory system, is an excellent herb to use.

Suggested dosage: ⅟₁₆–⅛ teaspoon per cup of water.

Warning: Be careful not to get it on your hands or, if you do, be sure to wash them thoroughly afterward. Before you know it you will rub your eyes or go to the bathroom and find yourself burning in whatever area you have touched.

Honey

Honey is the nectar of the flowers of plants, gathered by the bee, and stored in its stomach for transport to the hive. Plant nectars contain sucrose, water, amino acids, proteins, lipids, antioxidants, alkaloids, glycosides, thiamine, riboflavin, nicotinic acid, pantothenic acid, pyridoxine, biotin, folic acid, medoinositol, fumaric acid, succinic acid, oxalic acid, citric acid, tartaric acid, a-ketoglutaric acid, gluconic acid, glucuronic acid, allantoin, allantoic acid, dextrin, formic acid, a wide range of vitamins and minerals, and other unidentified compounds.

The sugar in plant nectars is primarily sucrose, a disaccharide. Sucrose (most commonly found in the form of white table sugar) is a double-molecule sugar, made from 1 fructose molecule and 1 glucose molecule linked together. When bees harvest plant nectars, they hold them in their stomachs for transport to the hive. During transport, their stomach enzymes break the sucrose molecule and apart into glucose and fructose. Glucose is slightly less sweet than sucrose; fructose is sweeter. Because fructose is so much sweeter than glucose and sucrose, it is a better food sweetener—it takes less calories to achieve the same level of sweetening produced by the other sugars.

When the bee arrives at the hive, it regurgitates the nectar into the wax cells of the honeycomb. The nectar is moved from cell to cell to facilitate drying. To hasten the process, large numbers of bees band together and fan their wings, facilitating the final evaporation that is necessary to thicken the nectar into what we call honey. At that point honey is about 80 percent solids and 20 percent liquid. Unlike sucrose, fructose and glucose in combination and at such a concentration are very stable. The fructose is the most stable and is very difficult to crystallize. When honey does crystallize, it usually is the glucose that is solid—the remaining liquid is primarily fructose. Fructose helps keep the honey liquid for extended periods of time. These two primary sugars of honey, glucose and fructose, are monosaccharides (simple sugars) and, as a result, do not require additional processing by the body to be digested. White sugar (a disaccharide) takes considerably more work to be digested. Other than plant fruits, honey, and the plant nectars it comes from, is the most ancient form of sugar concentrate the human species has used.

Historically, honeys came from a profusion of wildflowers, whatever grew locally. It was exceedingly uncommon to have a honey gathered from a single species of plant such as the alfalfa or clover honeys of today, unless that plant species existed in great abundance—heather is one notable exception. Because of this the honeys that humans have used throughout their evolutionary history have contained trace amounts of the medicinal compounds produced by a multitude of wild plants. Honey bees have a great attraction to many strongly medicinal plants: vitex, jojoba, elder, toadflax, balsam root, echinacea, valerian, dandelion, wild geranium—in fact almost any flowering medicinal herb, as well as the more commonly known alfalfas and clovers. The nectar from a multitude of medicinal plants is present in any wildflower honey mix.

These plant compounds, though present in tiny quantities, remain highly bioactive. This can be most easily seen in that honeys from poisonous plants can poison the people who eat them. Charles Millspaugh (1892) commented that the honey of Trebisond, produced from the Persian *Rhododendron ponticum*, is poisonous, as is honey produced from *Azalea pontica*. Ancient records have attributed at least one defeat of Roman soldiers to their having eaten poisonous honey the night before a battle. Even today beekeepers are warned to avoid allowing their bees to collect nectar from plants known to produce poisonous honey.

In addition to the plant nectar's individual medicinal qualities, the nectars are also subtly altered, in ways that modern science has been unable to explain, by their brief transport in the bees' digestive system. Before regurgitation the nectars combine in unique ways with the bees' digestive enzymes to produce new compounds.

Honey is not just another simple carbohydrate (like white sugar). It is composed of a highly complex collection of enzymes, plant pigments, organic acids, esters, antibiotic agents, and trace minerals. Honey, in fact, contains over 75 different compounds. Besides those already listed, it contains proteins, carbohydrates, hormones, and antimicrobial compounds. One pound of (non-heather) honey contains 1,333 calories (compared to white sugar at 1,748 calories), 1.4 g protein, 23 mg calcium, 73 mg phosphorus, 4.1 mg iron, 1 mg niacin, and 16 mg vitamin C. The content of each of these substances varies considerably, depending on what type of plants the honey is gathered from—some honey may contain as much as 300 mg vitamin C per 100 g of honey. Honey also contains vitamin A, beta-carotene, the complete complex of B vitamins, vitamin D, vitamin E, vitamin K, magnesium, sulphur, chlorine, potassium, iodine, sodium, copper, manganese, a rich supply of live enzymes, and relatively high concentrations of hydrogen peroxide. Many of the remaining substances in honey are so complex that they have yet to be identified. Honey has been found to possess antibiotic, antiviral, anti-inflammatory, anticarcinogenic, expectorant, antifungal, immune-stimulating, antiallergenic, laxative, antianemic, and tonic properties. Because honey increases calcium absorption in the body, it is also recommended during menopause to help prevent osteoporosis. In clinical trials honey has been found to be especially effective in treating stomach ulceration (especially that caused by *Helicobacter pylori* bacteria), infected wounds, severe skin ulceration, and respiratory illnesses. A Bulgarian study of 17,862 patients found that honey was effective in improving chronic bronchitis, asthmatic bronchitis, bronchial asthma, chronic and allergic rhinitis, and sinusitis.

Honey is a reliable, stable source of vitamins and minerals. Though high in vitamins, fruits and vegetables tend to lose them over time. Spinach, for instance, loses 50 percent of its vitamin C content within 24 hours of picking. Honey, on the other hand, stores its vitamins indefinitely. Wildflower honeys generally have the largest overall concentration of vitamins. Single-species honeys tend to increase concentrations of one vitamin to the detriment of others. For example, orange honey is relatively high in thiamine (8.2 mcg per 100 g), but low in nicotinic acid (0.16 mg per 100 g), while fireweed honey is low in thiamine (2.2 mcg) and high in nicotinic acid (0.86 mg). Though the levels may seem small, honey as a consistent addition to food has shown remarkable results in medical trials. Of one group of 58 boys, 29 were given 2 tablespoons of honey each day (one tablespoon in the morning and the other in the afternoon), and 29 none. All received the same diet, exercise, and rest. All were the same age and general health. The group receiving honey (after 1 year) showed an 8.5 percent increase in hemoglobin and an overall increase in vitality, energy,

> *Warning:* Occasionally, uncooked honeys can contain botulism spores that can be dangerous to children under 1 year old. The human digestive system is more developed and able to deactivate the spores after about age 1. In addition, in rare instances people who are allergic to bee stings or who have pollen sensitivity may react negatively to honey. If you have a history of allergic reactions, avoid honey.

and general appearance. Other studies in Switzerland and the United States echo these results. A number of modern researchers, in order to test the nutritional value of honey, have subsisted on diets of honey and milk for up to 3 months. In all cases they maintained their normal body weight and state of health.

Suggested dosage: 1 tablespoon per cup of tea. Generally raw, unprocessed, and unpasteurized wildflower honey should be used.

Single-plant honeys such as alfalfa and clover are generally from high-technology, monocropped fields that are doused with large amounts of pesticides and fertilizers. Use only organic wildflower honeys.

Maple Syrup (*Acer saccharinum*)

Sugar maple sap is virtually the only tree sap still used in the United States. Originally the Indians of North America, like many indigenous peoples, tapped not only all the maples (6 species) and birches (6 species) but also butternut and hickory trees. These saps were used not only as syrups—made by boiling them down—but as tonic drinks, that is, medicines.

Maple is rarely used in contemporary herbalism, but historically, during maple sap gathering, early New Englanders often drank the fresh sap as a primary spring tonic. (Now that I live in Vermont, I find that many maple sap harvesters still do.) Maple sap, and the syrup that comes from it, is one of the most complete nutrient foods known. It is possible to live for many weeks without any adverse physical effects eating only maple syrup. Maple syrup is high in calories, calcium, potassium, phosphorus, and vitamin B-12. It also contains significant amounts of many other B vitamins and iron. Maple sap has traditionally been used (internally and externally) as a general tonic; for skin conditions such as hives and stubborn wounds; as a kidney medicine, tonic, or diuretic; as a cough remedy; for cramping; and as a blood purifier.

Because of its complex nutritional makeup, its effectiveness as a general system tonic, and its impacts on the kidney system, maple syrup is especially useful when used on a long-term basis in fasting.

Suggested dosage: 2 tablespoons per 10 ounces of water—as often as desired daily.

Resources

WILDERNESS FASTING

Trishuwa
Foundation for Gaian Studies
505 Flint Road
Braintree, VT 05060
trishuwa@gaianstudies.org

RETREAT CENTER FASTING

Worldwide general list:
www.retreatsonline.com/guide/fasting.htm

British Columbia:
www.naturaldoc.com
1-800-661-5161

Arizona:
Tree of Life Rejuvenation Center
P.O. Box 1080
Patagonia, AZ 85624
1-520-394-2520
www.treeoflife.nu

California:
Fasting Center International (FCI)
www.fasting.com
1-805-899-4998

Portugal:
Moinhus Velhos
Cotifo
8600 Lagos
Portugal
Telephone: 351-282-687-147
www.juicefasting.com

MEDICAL FASTING FOR SERIOUS
DISEASE CONDITIONS

Joel Fuhrman, M.D.
Hunterdon Medical Center
Doctor's Office Building
1100 Wescott Drive, Suite 106
Flemington, NJ 08822
1-908-237-0200
www.drfuhrman.com

Notes

CHAPTER 1

[1]Kent Nerburn and Louise Mengelkoch, eds., *Native American Wisdom* (San Rafael, CA: New World Library, 1991), 43.

[2]James Hillman, *The Soul's Code* (New York: Random House, 1996), 41.

[3]Gloria Hutchinson, *A Retreat with Gerard Manley Hopkins and Hildegard of Bingen* (Cincinnati: St. Anthony Messenger Press, 1995), 42.

[4]M. K. Gandhi, *Fasting in Satyagraha* (Ahmedabad, India: Navajivan, 1965), 50.

[5]James Hillman, *The Thought of the Heart and the Soul of the World* (Woodstock, CT: Spring, 1995), 64.

CHAPTER 2

[1]Anthony Padovano, *A Retreat with Thomas Merton* (Cincinnati: St. Anthony Messenger Press, 1995), 57.

[2]Robert Bly, *News of the Universe* (San Francisco: Sierra Club Books, 1980), 211.

[3]Joan Halifax, *Shamanic Voices* (New York: Dutton, 1979), 6.

[4]Ibid., 6.

[5]Ibid., 1.

[6]Joseph Epes Brown, *The Sacred Pipe* (Norman: University of Oklahoma Press, 1953), 46.

[7]Quoted in Steven Foster and Meredith Little, *The Book of the Vision Quest* (New York: Prentice Hall, 1988), 24.

[8]Quoted in Margot Hellmiss and Norbert Kriegisch, *Healthy Fasting* (New York: Sterling, 1999), 30.

[9]Foster and Little, *The Book of the Vision Quest*, 24.

[10]William McNamara, *Mystical Passion* (Rockport, MA: Element Books, 1991), 97.

[11]Francis Densmore, *Teton Sioux Music* (Washington, D.C.: Smithsonian Institution, Bureau of American Ethnology, 1918), 188–89.

[12]Brown, *The Sacred Pipe*, 66.

[13]McNamara, *Mystical Passion*, 95.

[14]William McNamara, "The Desert and the City," *Desert Call* 29, 2/3 (summer/fall 1985), 21–22.

[15]Al-Ghazzali, *The Mysteries of Fasting*, translation by Nabih Amin Faris (Lahore: Sh. Muhammad Ashraf, 1987), 49.

[16]Quoted in Hellmiss and Kriegisch, *Healthy Fasting*, 16.

[17]M. K. Gandhi, *Fasting in Satyagraha* (Ahmedabad, India: Navajivan, 1965), 8.

[18]*Wisdom's Daughters* (New York: HarperCollins, 1993), 115.

[19]Ibid., 6.

[20]Al-Ghazzali, *The Mysteries of Fasting*, 49.

[21]Quoted in Shelley Kim Fines, *Spiritual Fasting* (Canada: Fines, 2001), 41.

[22]Ibid., 40.

[23]Gandhi, *Fasting in Satyagraha*, 22.

[24]Ibid., 24.

[25]Al-Ghazzali, *The Mysteries of Fasting*, 36.

[26]Gandhi, *Fasting in Satyagraha*, 52.

[27]Al-Ghazzali, *The Mysteries of Fasting*, 41.

[28]Gloria Hutchinson, *A Retreat with Gerard Manley Hopkins and*

Hildegard of Bingen (Cincinnati: St. Anthony Messenger Press, 1995), 27.

[29]Steven Foster and Meredith Little, commentary on fasting in wilderness.

[30]Halifax, *Shamanic Voices*, 13.

CHAPTER 3

[1]Carol Normandi and Laurelee Roark, *It's Not About Food* (New York: Perigee, 1999), 26.

[2]Geneen Roth, *When Food Is Love* (New York: Plume, 1992), 62.

[3]Ibid., 131.

CHAPTER 4

[1]Quoted in Carrie L'Esperance, *The Ancient Cookfire* (Santa Fe, NM: Bear, 1998), 5.

[2]Maria Linder, *Nutritional Biochemistry and Metabolism with Clinical Applications* (New York: McGraw Hill, 1991), 92.

[3]M. Bergendhal et al., "Homeostatic Joint Amplification of Pulsatile and 24-Hour Rhythmic Cortisol Secretion by Fasting Stress in Midluteal Phase Women: Concurrent Disruption of Cortisol-Growth Hormone, Cortisol-Luteinizing Hormone, and Cortisol-Leptin Synchrony," *J Clin Endocrinol Metab* 85, 11 (2000), 4028–35.

[4]Quoted in L'Esperance, *The Ancient Cookfire*, 5.

CHAPTER 5

[1]Carol Normandi and Laurelee Roark, *It's Not About Food* (New York: Perigee, 1999), 58–9.

[2]Ibid., 59.

[3]Kent Nerburn and Louise Mengelkoch, eds., *Native American Wisdom* (San Rafael, CA: New World Library, 1991), 35–6.

[4]Al-Ghazzali, *The Mysteries of Fasting* (Lahore: Sh. Muhammad Ashraf, 1987), 46.

[5]M. K. Gandhi, *Fasting in Satyagraha* (Ahmedabad, India: Navajivan, 1965), 17.

CHAPTER 6

[1]Quoted in Robert Bly, *The Winged Life* (San Francisco: Sierra Club Books, 1986), 7.

[2]Joseph Epes Brown, "The Question of 'Mysticism' within Native American Traditions," in *Understanding Mysticism*, edited by R. Woods (New York: Doubleday, 1980), 208.

[3]James Hillman, *The Thought of the Heart and the Soul of the World* (Woodstock, CT: Spring Publications, 1995), 37.

[4]Al-Ghazzali, *The Mysteries of Fasting* (Lahore: Sh. Muhammad Ashraf, 1987), 12.

[5]M. K. Gandhi, *Fasting in Satyagraha* (Ahmedabad, India: Navajivan, 1965), 76.

[6]Quoted in Stephen Harrod Buhner, *The Lost Language of Plants* (White River Junction, VT: Chelsea Green, 2002), 276.

[7]Dale Pendell, *Living with Barbarians* (Sebastopol, CA: Wild Ginger Press, 1999), 37–9.

[8]James Hillman, *The Thought of the Heart*, 63.

[9]Ibid., 66.

[10]Anthony Padovano, *A Retreat with Thomas Merton* (Cincinnati: St. Anthony Messenger Press, 1995), 19.

[11]Quoted in Carol Normandi and Laurelee Roark, *It's Not About Food* (New York: Perigee, 1999), 87.

[12]Geneen Roth, *When Food Is Love* (New York: Plume, 1992), 147.

References

BOOKS

* *An asterisk indicates: highly recommended.*

Paavo Airola. *How to Keep Slim, Healthy and Young with Juice Fasting.* Sherwood, OR: Health Plus, 2000.

Jane Alexander. *The Detox Plan.* Boston: Journey, 1998.

J. W. Armstrong. *The Water of Life.* Rustington, Sussex, England: True Health, n.d.

*Sidney MacDonald Baker. *Detoxification and Healing.* New Canaan, CT: Keats, 1997.

Francis Gano Benedict. *The Influence of Inanition on Metabolism.* Washington, D.C.: Carnegie Institute, 1907.

Peter Bennet and Stephen Barrie. *Seven-Day Detox Miracle.* New York: Prima, 2001.

*Robert Bly. *The Soul Is Here for Its Own Joy.* Hopewell, NJ: Ecco Press, 1995.

*Robert Bly. *The Winged Life.* San Francisco: Sierra Club Books, 1986.

*Robert Bly. *News of the Universe.* San Francisco: Sierra Club Books, 1980.

Paul Bragg. *The Miracle of Fasting.* Santa Barbara, CA: Health Science, n.d.

Nathaniel Hawthorn Bronner. *Quick Fasting.* Atlanta, GA: Century Systems, 2000.

Stanley Burroughs. *The Master Cleanser*. Kailua, HI: Burroughs, 1976.

Alan Cott. *Fasting, the Ultimate Diet*. Norwalk, CT: Hasting House, 1997.

Arnold Ehret. *Rational Fasting*. New York: Benedict Lust, 1971.

Bruce Fife. *The Detox Book*. Colorado Springs: HealthWise, 2001.

Shelley Kim Fines. *Spiritual Fasting*. Canada: Fines, 2001.

Joel Fuhrman. *Fasting and Eating for Health*. New York: St. Martin's Press, 1995.

M. K. Gandhi. *Fasting in Satyagraha*. Ahmedabad, India: Navajivan, 1965.

Al-Ghazzali. *The Mysteries of Fasting*. Lahore: Sh. Muhammad Ashraf, 1987.

Joan Halifax. *Shamanic Voices*. New York: Dutton, 1979.

John Heinerman. *Heinerman's Encyclopedia of Healing Juices*. Paramus, NJ: Reward Books, 1994.

Margot Hellmiss and Norbert Kriegisch. *Healthy Fasting*. New York: Sterling, 1999.

*James Hillman. *The Soul's Code*. New York: Random House, 1996.

*James Hillman. *The Thought of the Heart and the Soul of the World*. Woodstock, CT: Spring, 1995.

Gloria Hutchinson. *A Retreat with Gerard Manley Hopkins and Hildegard of Bingen*. Cincinnati: St. Anthony Messenger Press, 1995.

Carrie L'Esperance. *The Ancient Cookfire*. Santa Fe, NM: Bear, 1998.

Maria Linder. *Nutritional Biochemistry and Metabolism with Clinical Applications*. New York: McGraw Hill, 1991. Especially see chapter 8, "Nutrition and Metabolism of Protein," 87–109.

Steve Meyerowitz. *Juice Fasting and Detoxification*. Great Barrington, MA: Sproutman, 1999.

*Michael Murray. *The Complete Book of Juicing*. New York: Prima, 1998.

*Michael Murray and Joseph Pizzorno. *Textbook of Natural Medicine*. 2nd ed. Vol. 1. New York: Churchill Livingstone, 1999, 401–12. *NOTE:* this contains the best listing of research articles on therapeutic fasting in print.

Kent Nerburn and Louise Mengelkoch, eds. *Native American Wisdom*. San Rafael, CA: New World Library, 1991.

*Carol Normandi and Laurelee Roark. *It's Not About Food*. New York: Perigee, 1999.

Anthony Padovano. *A Retreat with Thomas Merton*. Cincinnati: St. Anthony Messenger Press, 1995.

*Geneen Roth. *When Food Is Love*. New York: Plume, 1992.

REVIEW ARTICLES ON THE PHYSIOLOGICAL EFFECTS OF FASTING

M. Bergendhal et al. "Homeostatic joint amplification of pulsatile and 24-hour rhythmic cortisol secretion by fasting stress in midluteal phase women: Concurrent disruption of cortisol-growth hormone, cortisol-luteinizing hormone, and cortisol-leptin synchrony." *J Clin Endocrinol Metab* 85(11) 2000, 4028–35.

M. Bergendahl et al. "Short-term fasting selectively suppresses leptin pulse mass and 24-hour rhythmic leptic release in healthy midluteal phase women without disturbing leptin pulse frequency or its entropy control (pattern orderliness)." *J Clin Endocrinol Metab* 85(1) 2000, 207–13.

D. A. Brouwer et al. "Influence of fasting on circulating levels of alpha-tocopherol and beta-carotene. Effect of short-term supplementation." *Clin Chim Acta* 277(2) Oct 1998, 127–39.

M. Cechowska-Pasko and J. Palka. "Age-dependent changes in glycosaminoglycan content in the skin of fasted rats: A possible mechanism." *Exp Toxicol Path* 52(2) 2000, 127–31.

M. Chechowska-Pasko and J. Palka. "Inhibition of collagen biosynthesis and increases in low molecular weight IGF-1 binding proteins in the skin of fasted rats." *Comp Biochem Physiol C Toxicol Pharmacol* 127(1) 2000, 49–59.

B. H. Chung et al. "Potencies of lipoproteins in fasting and post-prandial plasma to accept additional cholesterol molecules released from cell membranes." *Arteroscler Thromb Vasc Biol* 18(8) Aug 1998, 1217–30.

J. Dallongeville et al. "Short-term response of circulating leptin to feeding and fasting in man: Influence of circadian cycle." *Int J Obes Relat Metab Disord* 22(8) Aug 1998, 728–33.

S. M. Echwald et al. "Analysis of the relationship between fasting serum leptin levels and estimates of beta-cell function and insulin sensitivity in a population sample of 380 healthy young Caucasians." *Eur J Endocrinol* 140(2) Feb 1999, 180–5.

J. Fernandez and M. Valdeolmillos. "Increased levels of free fatty acids in fasted mice stimulate *in vivo* beta-cell electrical activity." *Diabetes* 47(11) Nov 1998, 1707–12.

A. Goldhamer et al. "Medically supervised water-only fasting in the treatment of hypertension." *J Manipulative Physiol* 24(5) 2001, 335–9.

W. R. Gower et al. "Regulation of atrial natriuretic peptide gene expression in gastric antrum by fasting." *Am J Physiol Regul Integr Comp Physiol* 278(3) 2000, R770–80.

K. Hojlund et al. "Reference intervals for glucose, beta-cell polypeptides, and counterregulatory factors during prolonged fasting." *Am J Physiol Endocrinol Metab* 280(1) 2001, E50–8.

T. J. Horton and J. O. Hill. "Prolonged fasting significantly changes nutrient oxidation and glucose tolerance after a normal mixed meal." *J Applied Physiology* 90(1) 2001, 155–63.

A. L. Kastin and V. Akerstrom. "Fasting, but not adrenalectomy, reduces transport of leptin into the brain." *Peptides* 21(5) 2000, 679–82.

L. E. Katz et al. "Dual regulation of insulin-like growth factor binding protein-1 levels by insulin and cortisol during fasting." *J Endocrinol Metab* 83(12) Dec 1998, 4426–30.

M. M. Kau et al. "Effects of fasting on aldosterone secretion in ovariectomized rats." *Chin J Physiol* 43(3) 2000, 125–30.

S. Kersten et al. "Characterization of the fasting-induced adipose factor FIAF, a novel peroxisome proliferator-activated receptor target gene." *J Biol Chem* 275(37) 2000, 28488–93.

Z. Kmiec et al. "The effects of fasting and refeeding on serum parathormone and calcitonin concentrations in young and old male rats." *Horm Metab Res* 33(5) 2001, 276–80.

I. Kowalska et al. "The effect of fasting and physical exercise on plasma leptin concentrations in high-fat fed rats." *J Physiol Pharmacol* 50(2) Jun 1999, 309–20.

N. La Paglia et al. "Leptin alters the response of the growth hormone releasing factor–growth hormone–insulin-like growth factor-1 axis to fasting." *J Endocrinol* 159(1) Oct 1998, 79–83.

T. C. Leone et al. "A critical role for the peroxisome proliferator-activated receptor alpha (PPARalpha) in the cellular fasting response: the PPARalpha-null mouse as a model of fatty acid oxidation disorders." *Proc Natl Acad Sci USA* 96(13) Jun 1999, 7473–8.

N. M. Lowe et al. "A comparison of the short-term kinetics of zinc metabolism in women during fasting and following a breakfast meal." *Br J Nutr* 80(4) Oct 1998, 363–70.

X. Y. Lu et al. "Differential distribution and regulation of OX1 and OX2 orexin/hypocretin receptor messenger RNA in the brain upon fasting." *Horm Behav* 37(4) 2000, 335–44.

M. Maccario et al. "Effects of 36-hour fasting on GH/IGF-1 axis and metabolic parameters in patients with simple obesity. Comparison with normal subjects and hypopituarity patients with severe GH deficiency." *Int J Obes Relat Metab Disord* 25(8) 2001, 1233–9.

M. Maccario et al. "Short-term fasting abolishes the sex-related differences in GH and leptin secretion in humans." *Am J Physiol Endocrinol Metab* 279(2) 2000, E411–6.

T. Mikami et al. "Alterations in the enzyme activity and protein contents of protein disulfide isomerase in rat tissues during fasting and refeeding." *Metabolism* 47 (9) Sept 1998, 1083–8.

H. Muller et al. "Fasting followed by vegetarian diet in patients with rheumatoid arthritis: A systematic review." *Scand J Rheumatol* 30(1) 2001, 1–10.

H. Norrelund et al. "The protein-retaining effects of growth hormone during fasting involve inhibition of muscle-protein breakdown." *Diabetes* 50(1) 2001, 96–104.

R. M. Ortiz et al. "Prolonged fasting increases the response of the renin-angiotensin-aldosterone system, but not vasopressin levels in postweaned northern elephant seal pups." *Gen Comp Endocrinol* 119(2) 2000, 217–23.

J. Peinado-Onsurbe et al. "Effect of fasting on hepatic lipase activity in the liver of developing rats." *Biol Neonate* 77(7) 2000, 131–8.

N. S. Rocha et al. "Effects of fasting and intermittent fasting on rat hepatocarcinogenesis induced by dimethylnitrosamine." *Teratog Carcinog Mutagen* 22(2) 2002, 129–38.

R. Roky et al. "Daytime alertness, mood, psychomotor performance, and oral temperature during Ramadan intermittent fasting." *Ann Nutr Metab* 44(3) 2000, 101–7.

E. J. Rolleman et al. "Changes in renal tri-iodothyronine and thyroxine handling during fasting." *Eur J Endocrinol* 142(2) 2000, 125–30.

H. Sogawa and C. Kubo. "Influence of short-term repeated fasting on the longevity of female F1 mice." *Mech Aging Dev* 115(1–2) 2000, 61–71.

J. F. Surmely et al. "Stimulation by leptin of 3H GDP binding to brown adipose tissue of fasted but not fed rats." *Int J Obes Relat Metab Disord* 22(9) Sep 1998, 923–6.

C. Thalhammer et al. "Endothelial cell dysfunction and arterial wall hypertrophy are associated with disturbed carbohydrate metabolism in patients at risk for cardiovascular disease." *Arterioscler Thromb Vasc Biol* 19(5) May 1999, 1173–9.

T. Tsuchiya et al. "Decrease of the obese gene expression in bovine subcutaneous adipose tissue by fasting." *Biosci Biotechnol Biochem* 62(10) Oct 1998, 2068–9.

K. A. van der Lee et al. "Fasting-induced changes in the expression of genes controlling substrate metabolism in the rat heart." *J Lipid Res* 42(11) 2001, 1752–8.

W. Vine et al. "Plasma amylin concentrations in fasted and fed rats quantified by a monoclonal immunoenzymometric assay." *Horm Metab Res* 30(9) Sep 1998, 581–5.

J. M. Weber and T. O'Connor. "Energy metabolism of the Virginia opossum during fasting and exercise." *J Exp Biol* 203 Pt 8 2000, 1365–71.

T. D. Williams et al. "Concurrent reductions in blood pressure and metabolic rate during fasting in the unrestrained SHR." *Am J Physiol Regul Integr Comp Physiol* 278(1) 2000, R255–62.

J. Zhang et al. "Reduction of hepatic insulin-like growth factor 1 (IGF-1) messenger ribonucleic acid (mRNA) during fasting is associated with diminished splicing of IGF-1 pre-mRNA and decreased stability of cytoplasmic IGF-1 mRNA." *Endocrinology* 139(11) Nov 1998, 4523–30.

Index

About the Author

Stephen Harrod Buhner is a master herbalist, a psychotherapist, and an expert on indigenous and contemplative spiritual traditions. He has been interested in the health benefits of fasting for over 30 years; for the past two decades, he and his wife Trishuwa, a metis of Cherokee and Irish ancestry, have been leading wilderness fasting retreats. Stephen's work and writing focus on herbal and alternative healing, deep ecology, and sacred plant medicine. He lives in Vermont.